5 Ingredient Ketogenic Diet Cookbook

113 Easy 5 Ingredient Keto Diet Recipes For Quick Meals And Rapid Weight Loss

FREDA DAVIS

Copyright © 2018 Freda Davis

All rights reserved. No part of this publication may be reproduced, distributed, or transmitted in any form or by any means, including photocopying, recording, or other electronic or mechanical methods, without the prior written permission of the publisher, except in the case of brief quotations embodied in critical reviews and certain other noncommercial uses permitted by copyright law.

Limit of Liability/Disclaimer of Warranty: While the publisher and author have used their best efforts in preparing this book, they make no representations or warranties with respect to the accuracy or completeness of the contents of this book and specifically disclaim any implied warranties of merchantability or fitness for a particular purpose. No warranty may be created or extended by sales representatives or written sales materials. The advice and strategies contained herein may not be suitable for your situation. You should consult with a professional where appropriate. Neither the publisher nor author shall be liable for any loss of profit or any other commercial damages, including but not limited to special, incidental, consequential, or other damages.

ISBN-13: 978-1723166754
ISBN-10: 1723166758

DEDICATION

To diligent homemakers all over the world!

TABLE OF CONTENT

INTRODUCTION 1

BREAKFAST.. 5

    Creamy Scrambled Eggs (Stove top) 5

    Cheddar Mushroom Omelet (Stove top)................................. 6

    Cottage Cheese Egg Salad (Stove top).................................... 7

    Egg Sausage Casserole (Oven) 8

    Microwave Keto Bread (Microwave)...................................... 9

    Almond Flour Biscuits (Oven)... 11

    Bacon, Eggs And Avocado (Stove top).................................. 12

    Eggs And Asparagus (Stove top).. 13

    Sausage And Bell Pepper Stir Fry (Stove top)....................... 15

    Creamy Bacon And Tomatoes (Stove top) 16

    Eggs And Herbs (Stove top) 17

    Herbed Feta Cheese Omelet (Stove top) 18

    Everyday Cream Cheese Pancakes (Stove top) 19

    Skillet Ground Turkey And Eggs (Stove top)........................ 20

VEGETABLE AND SALAD 22

    Roasted Cauliflower Bites (Oven) 22

    Baked Cauliflower Salad (Oven).. 23

    Cheddar And Broccoli Soup (Stove top) 24

    Easy Spinach Bake (Oven) 25

    Mushroom And Vegetables (Stove top) 27

    Zucchini Noodles With Tomatoes And Olives (Stove top) 28

Roasted Radish With Basil (Oven) 29

Green Bean And Almond Salad (Stove top) 30

Zucchini Scrambled Eggs (Stove top) 31

Cheesy Zucchini And Eggplant (Slow cooker) 33

SOUP AND STEW 34

Coconut Curry (Stove top) 34

Delicious Cauliflower Soup (Stove top) 35

Dried Vegetable Soup (Stove top) 36

Bell Pepper Soup (Stove top) 37

Creamy Pumpkin Soup (Stove top) 39

Coconut Chicken Curry (Slow cooker) 40

Zucchini And Herbs Soup (Stove top) 41

Easy Celery Soup (Oven) 42

Chicken Endives Soup (Stove top) 43

Easiest Onion Soup (Stove top) 44

POULTRY MAIN DISH 46

Easiest Baked Chicken Breasts (Oven) 46

Rosemary Chicken And Bacon (Grill) 47

Creamy Ranch Chicken (Oven) 48

Prosciutto Chicken Breast (Oven) 50

Easy Turkey Burgers (Grill) 51

Chicken Breasts With Spinach Pesto (Oven) 52

Teriyaki Chicken (Grill) 53

Marinated Garlic Chicken (Grill) 54

Garlic Turkey Thighs (Slow cooker) 55

Juicy Pepper Chicken (Stove top) 56

Cheesy Stuffed Chicken Breasts (Oven) 58

Marinated Grilled Chicken (Grill) 59

Slow Cooked Creamy Chicken (Slow cooker) 60

Chicken Garam Masala (Stove top) 61

Chicken Salsa Verde (Oven) 62

Turkey Legs (Oven) 63

BEEF MAIN DISH 65

Good Time Rib Roast (Oven) 65

Delightful Pot Roast (Slow cooker) 67

Juicy Prime Rib Roast (Oven) 68

Balsamic Filet Mignon (Stove top) 69

Garlic Butter Sirloin Steak (Grill) 71

Creamy Beef On Toast (Stove top) 72

Family Beef Tenderloin 73

Tender Beef Roast (Slow cooker) 74

Everyday Roast Beef 75

Salty Prime Rib Roast (Oven) 76

Grilled Hamburgers (Grill) 77

BBQ Beef Brisket (Oven) 78

Easiest Cube Steaks 79

Poblano Pot Roast (Slow cooker) 80

Spicy Burgers (Grill) 81

Spinach Meatloaf (Oven) 82

PORK MAIN DISH 84

Parmesan Pork Chops (Oven) 84

Ham And Leeks (Oven) 85

Quick Pork Chops (Stove top) 86

Spicy Pork Tenderloin (Oven, Stove top) 88

Stir Fry Pork Chops (Stove top) 89

Glazed Pulled Pork (Slow cooker) 90

Almond Flour Coated Pork Chops (Stove top) 92

Cheesy Skillet Pork Chops (Stove top) 93

Teriyaki Pork Kebabs (Grill) 94

Chorizo Made At Home 95

Spicy Sausage Patties (Stove top) 96

Omelet With Ground Pork (Stove top) 97

SEAFOOD MAIN DISH 99

Cajun Grilled Shrimp (Grill) 99

Quick Tomato Salmon (Oven) 100

Weeknight Trout (Oven) 101

Cheesy Salmon (Oven) 103

Cheesy Grilled Cod (Grill) 104

Oven Fried Shrimp (Oven) 105

Greek Style Tilapia (Oven) 106

Easy Baked Halibut (Oven) 108

Lemon Pepper Rosemary Cod (Oven) 109

Easy Baked Halibut (Oven) 110

SIDE DISH 112

Mushroom Soup (Stove top) 112

Crispy Kale Chips (Oven) 113

Sautéed Bok Choy (Stove Top) 114

Lemon Cauliflower "Rice" (Microwave) 115

Roasted Cabbage (Oven) 117

Keto Mashed Cauliflower (Stove top) 118

Roasted Broccoli (Oven) 119

Easy Cucumber Salad 120

Mushroom Stir Fry (Stove top) 121

Cabbage Stir Fry (Stove top) 123

Zucchini Chips (Oven) 124

Sautéed Collard Greens (Stove top) 125

Roasted Mushrooms And Asparagus (Oven) 126

Roasted Tomato And Eggplant (Oven) 127

Tomato Ginger Salad 128

Easiest Roasted Salmon (Oven) 129

DESSERT / FAT BOMB 130

Peanut Butter Cookies (Oven) 130

Chocolate Peanut Butter Cookies (Oven) 132

Egg-Free Chocolate Mousse 133

Coconut Balls Fat Bomb (Stove top) 134

Chocolate Fat Bombs (Stove top) 135

Creamy Chocolate Frosty 136

Keto Flan Cups (Oven) 137

Easy Chocolate Pudding 138

Almond Butter Cookies (Oven) 139

INTRODUCTION

Meals don't have to be boring because you are on a diet. The keto lifestyle can be exciting when you have a collection of recipes that you can cook very easily and very quickly. Gone are the days when quick and easy means you have to compromise on taste. The recipes in the *5 Ingredient Ketogenic Diet Cookbook* have suffered no compromise whatsoever in taste and palate satisfaction. They are innovative, delicious and fabulous! And your pantry already has most of the ingredients that you need with the addition of just a few extras.

This book adopts the principle of "less is more". By focusing on true taste, you can use fewer ingredients to make dishes that are healthy and full of flavor. Whether it is breakfast, lunch or weeknight dinner, cooking keto meals have never been this stress-free. The incredibly short shopping list and easy to find ingredients will save you a lot of time whenever you need to restock your pantry.

Get a head start on eating healthy by planning your meals in advance. The 113 recipes in this book are designed to make things easier for you. Nutritional information is also clearly provided as a further guide. Browse the categories and choose what you will be cooking for the week. Then you can look through your pantry to know the ingredients you already have and the few items you may have to buy. These recipes use everyday ingredients that you cook with regularly. They are easy to find and very affordable.

No limitation is placed on style of cooking. Each recipe is clearly labeled according to the appliance that is required for making the dish. So, apart from selecting the recipes that appeal to you, you can also easily know whether to get your oven ready or bring out a skillet or saucepan. A good number of these meals are made with a slow cooker for those who love the time saving and minimal hands on time slow cooking provides. If you love grilling, your grill will become a quick way to get diner ready with more than 10 easy grilling recipes in this collection.

There is no need to go to a restaurant for dinner when you can cook great tasting *Creamy Ranch Chicken* right in your own kitchen. Get the best flavored chicken breast with just a few ingredients. It cooks easily in the oven to give you juicy baked chicken breasts for a sumptuous, restaurant-style dinner. The butter and parmesan cheese create the perfect combination of melt-in-your-mouth flavor. *Quick Pork Chops* is a simple to cook recipe that comes out juicy and tender. Soy sauce and apple cider vinegar come together with garlic to make a delightful weeknight dish. You will savor every bite of this delicious combination.

Rice and other grains have to be discarded when you go keto but cauliflower comes to the rescue. Not only does it stand in for rice, it also provides a good substitute for mashed potatoes. *The Lemon Cauliflower "Rice"* recipe comes together in a few minutes and lets you have a good side dish that can go with most meat and fish main dishes. *Keto Mashed Cauliflower* provides a good stand in whenever you need mashed potatoes.

When you place the *Teriyaki Chicken* on the dinner table, your family will think you spent the whole in the kitchen, but you and I know the marinade has only two ingredients! A cup of mayonnaise and 3/4 cup of soy sauce is all that is required to create this fabulous Asian flavor. The 30 minutes marinating time allows that flavor to seep deep into the meat. Roasting on a grill adds a smoky flavor that you can't get in an oven.

These and much more await you in the *5 Ingredient Ketogenic Diet Cookbook*. Don't wait any longer, dig in and start cooking the mot fabulous ketogenic meals!

Freda Davis

4

BREAKFAST

Creamy Scrambled Eggs (Stove top)
Soft, creamy and wholesome breakfast.

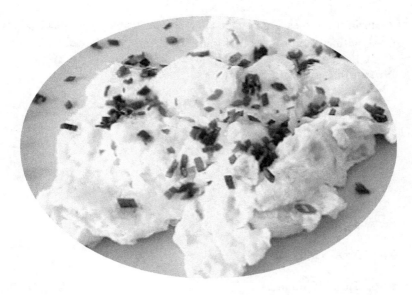

Servings: 2

Prep Time: 5 minutes

Cook Time: 5 minutes

Ingredients:

4 eggs, beaten

1 tablespoon butter

1/4 cup cottage cheese

1 teaspoon chopped fresh chives

Ground black pepper, to taste

Directions:

1. In a skillet, melt the butter on medium heat. Pour in the eggs then cook for 1 to 2 minutes.

2. Stir in the chives and cottage cheese then sprinkle with black pepper. Cook with stirring for about 4 minutes, or until eggs are almost set.

Nutrition Guide Per Serving:

Calories 234, Carbs 1.9g, Protein 16.3g, Fat 17g

Cheddar Mushroom Omelet (Stove top)

Servings: 2

Prep Time: 5 minutes

Cook Time: 10 minutes

Ingredients:

2 handfuls button mushrooms, sliced

2 tablespoons olive oil

1 large handful parsley leaves, chopped roughly

1/2 cup grated cheddar cheese

4 eggs, beaten

Directions:

1. Heat olive oil in a large skillet on medium heat. Add the mushrooms and cook with occasional stirring for 2 to 3 minutes. Transfer to a bowl and toss with parsley and cheese.

2. Add the eggs to the remaining oil in the pan. Cook until set, swirling occasionally with a fork.

3. Scoop the mushroom mixture over one side of the omelet then flip over the other half of the omelet to cover the mixture. Cook for a couple of minutes more. Serve.

Nutrition Guide Per Serving:

Calories 390, Carbs 0.3g, Protein 23g, Fat 33g

Cottage Cheese Egg Salad (Stove top)

Servings: 2

Prep Time: 5 minutes

Cook Time: 15 minutes

Ingredients:

4 hard-boiled eggs

2/3 cup 1% cottage cheese

Seasoned salt and pepper, to taste

Dash of paprika

Directions:

1. Hard boil the eggs then remove the shells,

2. Chop eggs on a plate and mix with cottage cheese. Season to taste.

Nutrition Guide Per Serving:

Calories 149, Carbs 2.8g, Protein 19.2g, Fat 6.3g

Egg Sausage Casserole (Oven)
A simple and filling breakfast.

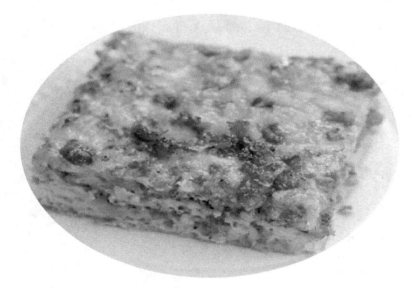

Servings: 12

Prep Time: 10 minutes

Cook Time: 30 minutes

Ingredients:

12 large eggs

12 ounces breakfast sausage, browned

2 cups shredded low-fat Cheddar cheese

1/4 cup coconut milk

1/4 teaspoon pepper

Directions:

1. Preheat your oven to 375°F. Grease a casserole dish.

2. Mix together all the ingredients and pour into the dish.

3. Bake in a the oven for 30 minutes. Let cool for 5 minutes before serving.

Nutrition Guide Per Serving:

Calories 200, Carbs 2.1g, Protein 15.8g, Fat 34.8g

Microwave Keto Bread (Microwave)

Servings: 2

Prep Time: 1 minutes

Cook Time: 1 minute 30 seconds

Ingredients:

1/4 cup almond flour

1 tablespoon coconut flour

1 large egg

1 teaspoon coconut oil

1/4 teaspoon baking powder

Directions:

1. Mix all the ingredients together then scoop into a ramekin or mug.

2. Microwave for 90 seconds then remove.

3. Turn over onto a plate (you may have to run a knife around the edges).

4. Slice into 2 and serve.

Nutrition Guide Per Serving:

Calories 167, Carbs 7.3g, Protein 7.4g, Fat 13g

Almond Flour Biscuits (Oven)

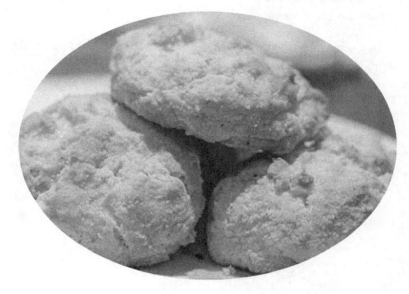

Servings: 12

Prep Time: 10 minutes

Cook Time: 12 minutes

Ingredients:

3 cups almond flour

4 tablespoons salted butter

4 large eggs, beaten

2/3 cup sour cream

2 teaspoon baking powder

Directions:

1. Preheat your oven to 400°F. Grease 12 muffin tins.

2. Melt butter in a saucepan then remove from heat. Add eggs and sour cream and stir to combine.

3. In a bowl, mix together almond flour and baking powder. Stir the dry ingredients into the wet

until you have a dough.

4. Divide the dough into 12 muffin tins.

5. Bake until the tops start to turn brown, about 12 minutes.

Nutrition Guide Per Serving:

Calories 265, Carbs 4.8g, Protein 10g, Fat 23g

Bacon, Eggs And Avocado (Stove top)

Servings: 2

Prep Time: 5 minutes

Cook Time: 10 minutes

Ingredients:

4 strips of bacon

1 large ripe avocado, peeled, sliced

2 large eggs

1/2 teaspoon seasoned salt

Juice from 1/2 a lime

Directions:

1. Add the bacon and avocado to a skillet on medium heat. Cook for about 3 minutes then flip and cook for 1 minute. Transfer to a plate, sprinkle with seasoned salt and drizzle with lime juice then set aside.

2. Crack the eggs into the drippings in the pan. Fry for about 2 minutes then flip and fry until done.

3. Serve eggs with bacon and avocado.

Nutrition Guide Per Serving:

Calories 312, Carbs 2.6g, Protein 13g, Fat 27g

Eggs And Asparagus (Stove top)
Just 20 minutes and breakfast is ready for two.

Servings: 2

Prep Time: 5 minutes

Cook Time: 15 minutes

Ingredients:

10 - 12 asparagus stalks, trimmed

2 teaspoons olive oil

4 eggs

1/4 cup grated Parmesan cheese

Salt and pepper to taste

Directions:

1. Heat the olive oil in skillet on medium heat. Add the asparagus and toss with a little salt. Cook for 4 to 5 minutes, or until the asparagus is tender.

2. Spread out the asparagus then crack the eggs over. Sprinkle with Parmesan, reduce to low heat and cover. Allow the eggs to cook for 10 to 12 minutes , or until done to your liking.

3. Serve sprinkled with pepper.

Nutrition Guide Per Serving:

Calories 305, Carbs 2.4g, Protein 20g, Fat 25g

Sausage And Bell Pepper Stir Fry (Stove top)
A delicious, no-hassle breakfast.

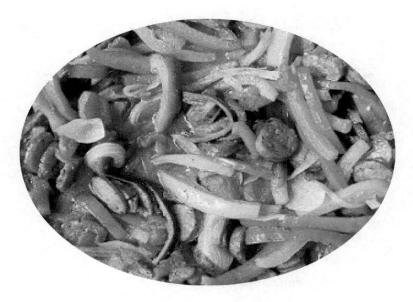

Servings: 4

Prep Time: 5 minutes

Cook Time: 10 minutes

Ingredients:

1 pound turkey sausage, sliced

2 teaspoons vegetable oil

1 large bell pepper (red or green)

1/2 red onion, sliced

1/4 cup shredded mild cheddar cheese

Directions:

1. Heat oil in a large skillet on medium heat. Add the sausage and cook for about 3 minutes.

2. Add the rest of the ingredients and cook until vegetables are softened and sausage is browned.

3. Sprinkle with cheese and let melt before removing from heat. Serve.

Nutrition Guide Per Serving:

Calories 328, Carbs 5g, Protein 30g, Fat 21g

Creamy Bacon And Tomatoes (Stove top)

Servings: 2

Prep Time: 5 minutes

Cook Time: 5 minutes

Ingredients:

4 slices cured bacon

2 large red tomatoes

1/2 cup, shredded cheddar cheese

I teaspoon of water

Directions:

1. Add the bacon to a skillet on medium heat. Sauté until browned.

2. Add the tomato and water then sprinkle with cheese. Cover and let heat through until cheese melts, about 1 to 2 minutes.

3. Serve.

Nutrition Guide Per Serving:

Calories 235, Carbs 6.2g, Protein 21g, Fat 13.9g

Eggs And Herbs (Stove top)

Servings: 4

Prep Time: 4 minutes

Cook Time: 6 minutes

Ingredients:

1 1/2 tablespoons of unsalted butter

4 eggs

2 tablespoons water

1/2 cup of chopped mixed fresh herbs (such as cilantro, parsley)

Salt and freshly ground black pepper, to taste

Directions:

1. Add butter to a skillet on medium heat.

2. Whisk together eggs and water. Seasoned to taste with salt and pepper. Pour into the hot butter and cook with occasional stirring for about 4 to 5 minutes, or until done to your liking.

3. Stir in the herbs.

Nutrition Guide Per Serving:

Calories 184, Carbs 1.5g, Protein 13g, Fat 13.7g

Herbed Feta Cheese Omelet (Stove top)

Servings: 2

Prep Time: 5 minutes

Cook Time: 5 minutes

Ingredients:

6 eggs, beaten

Kosher salt and black pepper, to taste

2 tablespoon of chopped herbs, (such as basil, parsley)

2 tablespoon of unsalted butter

4 ounces crumbled feta cheese

Directions:

1. Whisk the eggs with salt and pepper to taste.

2. In a large skillet, melt the butter on medium heat. Add the eggs and cook for about 3 to 4 minutes or until just set.

3. Sprinkle the cheese on top of the eggs then fold into half. Let cook for about 1 minute, or until cheese melts.

Nutrition Guide Per Serving:

Calories 520, Carbs 3g, Protein 31g, Fat 43g

Everyday Cream Cheese Pancakes (Stove top)
Very light and creamy pancakes.

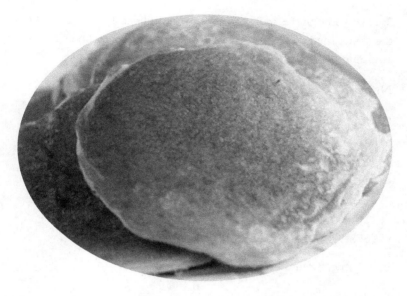

Servings: 2

Prep Time: 5 minutes

Cook Time: 8 minutes

Ingredients:

2 1/2 ounces cream cheese

2 eggs

1/2 tablespoon butter

1 tablespoon coconut flakes

1 teaspoon cinnamon

Directions:

1. Combine eggs and cream cheese in a bowl then whisk until creamy. Stir in coconut flakes and cinnamon.

2. Heat some butter in a skillet on medium heat. Pour half of the batter into the skillet then cook for 2 minutes, or until golden. Flip and cook for about 1 minute on the other side. Repeat with the remaining batter.

Nutrition Guide Per Serving:

Calories 439, Carbs 2.8g, Protein 18g, Fat 41g

Skillet Ground Turkey And Eggs (Stove top)

Servings: 2

Prep Time: 5 minutes

Cook Time: 15 minutes

Ingredients:

1 pound ground turkey

1 cup salsa

6 eggs

Oil

Directions:

1. Coat the bottom of a skillet with some oil and place on medium heat. Add turkey then cook and stir until browned.

2. Stir in the salsa and cook for about 3 minutes.

3. Crack eggs over the mixture then cover and cook until egg whites are done, about 5 to 7 minutes.

Nutrition Guide Per Serving:

Calories 390, Carbs 3g, Protein 41g, Fat 22g

VEGETABLE AND SALAD

Roasted Cauliflower Bites (Oven)

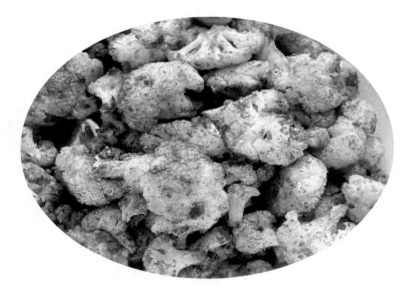

Servings: 4

Prep Time: 10 minutes

Cook Time: 40 minutes

Ingredients:

1 head cauliflower, cut into florets

1/4 teaspoon of garlic powder

2 tablespoons of extra-virgin olive oil

1/2 cup grated Parmesan

Salt and ground black pepper, to taste

Directions:

1. Preheat your oven to 400°F.

2. Add the cauliflower florets to a rimmed baking sheet. Drizzle with olive oil then sprinkle with salt, pepper and garlic powder.

3. Roast n the oven, tossing occasionally for 30 minutes. Add the Parmesan, tossing to combine then roast for 10 minutes longer.

Nutrition Guide Per Serving:

Calories 96, Carbs 7.6g, Protein 3g, Fat 6.8g

Baked Cauliflower Salad (Oven)

Servings: 6

Prep Time: 10 minutes

Cook Time: 30 minutes

Ingredients:

1 large head cauliflower, cut into florets

1 tablespoon tahini

1 cup Greek yoghurt

2 tablespoons currants

1 bunch mint, leaves picked

Directions:

1. Preheat your oven to 400°F. Line a baking sheet with aluminum foil.

2. Arrange cauliflower florets on the baking sheet, spray with cooking oil then sprinkle with a little salt and pepper.

3. Roast with occasional turning for 25 minutes, or until the cauliflower is tender.

4. Sprinkle with the currants then roast for additional 5 minutes.

5. In the meantime, mix together tahini and yogurt in a serving platter. Top with the roasted cauliflower and garnish with mint leaves.

Nutrition Guide Per Serving:

Calories 80, Carbs 10g, Protein 7g, Fat 2g

Cheddar And Broccoli Soup (Stove top)

Servings: 4

Prep Time: 5 minutes

Cook Time: 25 minutes

Ingredients:

2 cups chopped broccoli

1 3/4 cups chicken broth

2 cups heavy whipping cream

1 teaspoon garlic powder

1 1/2 cup shredded cheddar cheese

Directions:

1. In a large pot, combine all the ingredients except cheddar cheese.

2. Bring to a boil on medium high heat then reduce the heat and let simmer for 20 minutes.

3. Stir in the cheese and let cook until it melts.

Nutrition Guide Per Serving:

Calories 249, Carbs 4.4g, Protein 12.5g, Fat 25g

Easy Spinach Bake (Oven)

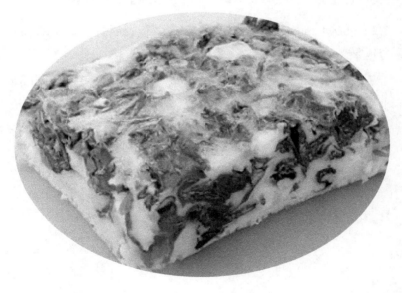

Servings: 8

Prep Time: 15 minutes

Cook Time: 10 minutes

Ingredients:

10 ounces frozen chopped spinach, thawed

1 garlic clove, crushed

4 eggs, beaten

Salt and pepper, to taste

Directions:

1. Preheat your oven to 350°F. Line a rimmed 9x13 baking sheet with non-stick paper

2. Squeeze the spinach to remove as much water as possible.

3. In a bowl, mix the spinach with garlic and eggs. Season with salt and pepper.

4. Scoop the mixture into the prepared baking sheet. Bake until firm and springy, about 10-15 minutes.

5. Remove from oven and let cool in the tin before cutting. Serve, topped with cream cheese.

Nutrition Guide Per Serving:

Calories 48, Carbs 2.3g, Protein 4.1g, Fat 2.7g

Mushroom And Vegetables (Stove top)

You can serve this with cauliflower rice and soy sauce.

Servings: 4

Prep Time: 15 minutes

Cook Time: 15 minutes

Ingredients:

4 large Portobello mushroom caps

1 tablespoon olive oil

1 green bell pepper, sliced

1 onion, sliced

3 garlic cloves, minced

Directions:

1. Heat the oil in a skillet on medium heat. Add the onion, garlic and bell pepper. Cook for about 5 minutes then season with a little salt.

2. Add the mushroom caps, reduce to low heat, cover then cook until mushrooms are tender, about 10 minutes. Flip once after 5 minutes.

Nutrition Guide Per Serving:

Calories 80, Carbs 10g, Protein 3.5g, Fat 3.8g

Zucchini Noodles With Tomatoes And Olives (Stove top)

Servings: 4

Prep Time: 15 minutes

Cook Time: 5 minutes

Ingredients:

1/3 cup sun dried tomato pesto

4 medium sized zucchini, julienned

1/3 cup halved pitted kalamata olives

1/2 pint cherry tomatoes

1/2 cup grated parmesan cheese

Directions:

1. Heat the pesto in large skilled on medium-high heat.

2. Add the julienned zucchini and cook for 2 minutes.

3. Add the olives and tomatoes then cook for additional 2 minutes.

4. Top with the cheese and toss to coat. Serve.

Nutrition Guide Per Serving:

Calories 116, Carbs 9.8g, Protein 7.5g, Fat 6g

Roasted Radish With Basil (Oven)

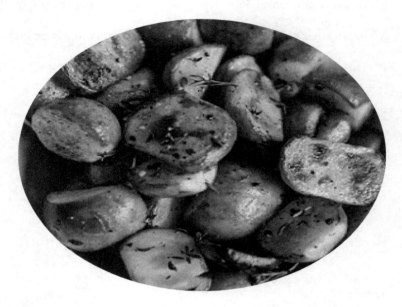

Servings: 6

Prep Time: 5 minutes

Cook Time: 35 minutes

Ingredients:

3 bunches radishes

2 teaspoons fresh basil, chopped

1 tablespoon coconut oil, melted

2 teaspoons lemon juice

Salt and pepper, to taste

Directions:

1. Wash the radishes and cut them into quarters.

2. Preheat your oven to 350°F and place parchment paper on a sheet pan.

3. Mix together coconut oil, radishes, salt and pepper in a large bowl.

4. Transfer radishes to the sheet pan and roast for 35 minutes. Stir once or twice.

5. Serve, tossed with basil and lemon juice.

Nutrition Guide Per Serving:

Calories 39, Carbs 4.5g, Protein 1g, Fat 3g

Green Bean And Almond Salad (Stove top)

Servings: 8

Prep Time: 10 minutes

Cook Time: 25 minutes

Ingredients:

2 pounds fresh green beans, trimmed

1/2 cup sliced almonds

2 tablespoons of balsamic vinegar

1/2 cup olive oil

Directions:

1. Cover the beans with water in a saucepan. Bring to a boil and cook for about 15 minutes. Transfer to cold water to cool for a few minutes then drain.

2. In a large bowl, combine green beans with balsamic vinegar and olive oil.

3. Place a skillet on low heat and add the almonds. Cook until light brown.

4. Add almonds to the green beans and toss.

Nutrition Guide Per Serving:

Calories 194, Carbs 9.7g, Protein 3.2g, Fat 17g

Zucchini Scrambled Eggs (Stove top)

Servings: 2

Prep Time: 5 minutes

Cook Time: 7 minutes

Ingredients:

1 medium zucchini, sliced

1 tablespoon olive oil

2 eggs, beaten

1 garlic clove, minced

Salt and pepper, to taste

Directions:

1. Heat oil in a medium skillet on medium heat. Add garlic then cook and stir for 1 minute. Add the zucchini and cook until softened.

2. Spread the zucchini in a single layer then pour the eggs on top. Cook until the eggs are firm.

3. Season with salt and pepper and serve.

Nutrition Guide Per Serving:

Calories 185, Carbs 4.5g, Protein 7g, Fat 15.7g

Cheesy Zucchini And Eggplant (Slow cooker)

Servings: 8

Prep Time: 20 minutes

Cook Time: 2 hours 30 minutes

Ingredients:

1 medium zucchini, cut into bite size pieces

1 medium eggplant, peeled, cut into bite size pieces

1 medium onion, sliced

2/3 cup shredded Parmesan cheese, divided

1 1/2 cups light spaghetti sauce

Directions:

1. Add the zucchini, eggplant, onion, 1/3 cup of the shredded Parmesan cheese and the spaghetti sauce to a 4-quart slow cooker

2. Cover then cook for 4 to 5 hours on Low heat or 2 to 2-1/2 hours on High heat.

3. Sprinkle with the reserved Parmesan cheese when you serve.

Nutrition Guide Per Serving:

Calories 54, Carbs 9g, Protein 3.2g, Fat 1.3g

SOUP AND STEW

Coconut Curry (Stove top)

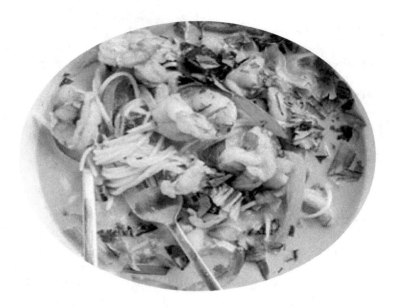

Servings: 2

Prep Time: 10 minutes

Cook Time: 10 minutes

Ingredients:

3 tablespoons Thai green curry paste

1 1/2 cups coconut milk

1 large Zucchini, julienned

5 - 6 ounces cooked shrimp

Cooking oil

Directions:

1. Heat a little oil in skillet on medium heat. Stir in the curry paste and cook for just 1 minute.

2. Add the coconut milk, let come to a boil then let cook for a few minutes.

3. Add the Zucchini and prawns. Cook for 1 to 2 minutes then remove from heat.

Nutrition Guide Per Serving:

Calories 477, Carbs 10g, Protein 18g, Fat 39g

Delicious Cauliflower Soup (Stove top)
Very simple soup made with pureed cauliflower.

Servings: 4

Prep Time: 10 minutes

Cook Time: 10 minutes

Ingredients:

1 head cauliflower, cut into florets

1 quart of water

Salt and pepper, to taste

1 tablespoon unsalted butter

Grated Parmesan cheese, for topping

Directions:

1. In a large saucepan, combine the water with 2 teaspoons of salt and bring to a boil. Add the cauliflower and cook for 5 to 7 minutes or until very soft.

2. Drain the cauliflower but reserve the cooking water.

3. Add half of the cauliflower, 1/2 tablespoon of butter and some of the cooking water to a blender. Blend until smooth, adding more of the cooking water as necessary to achieve soup consistency.

4. Repeat with the remaining cauliflower.

Nutrition Guide Per Serving:

Calories 58, Carbs 10.5g, Protein 4.5g, Fat 3g

Dried Vegetable Soup (Stove top)

Servings: 4

Prep Time: 5 minutes

Cook Time: 5 minutes

Ingredients:

1/3 cup dried soup vegetables

4 cups chicken stock

2 tablespoons of coconut oil, melted

Ground black pepper, to taste

Sea salt, to taste

Directions:

1. In a large saucepan mix all the ingredients together.

2. Bring to a boil on medium heat then let cook for 1 to 2 minutes.

3. Remove from heat and serve.

Nutrition Guide Per Serving:

Calories 125, Carbs 2.3g, Protein 2.7g, Fat 11.6g

Bell Pepper Soup (Stove top)

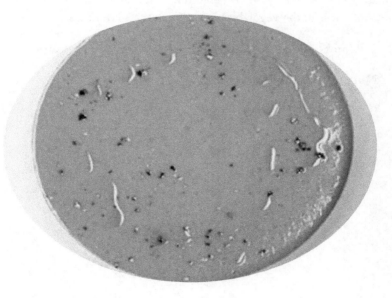

Servings: 4

Prep Time: 15 minutes

Cook Time: 35 minutes

Ingredients:

1 pound red bell peppers, seeded, sliced

1 large bunch fresh basil, chopped

5 garlic cloves, sliced

1 cup heavy cream

1 teaspoon sea salt

Directions:

1. In a large saucepan mix all the ingredients together.

2. Cover, bring to a boil on medium heat then reduce to a simmer and let cook until all the vegetables are soft, about 30 minutes.

3. Remove from the heat and process in a blender until smooth.

Nutrition Guide Per Serving:

Calories 227, Carbs 6.6g, Protein 2.1g, Fat 22g

Creamy Pumpkin Soup (Stove top)

Servings: 4

Prep Time: 10 minutes

Cook Time: 35 minutes

Ingredients:

2 cups vegetable stock

2 cups roasted pumpkin

1 teaspoon of onion powder

Salt and pepper, to taste

1/2 cup of heavy cream

Directions:

1. In a large saucepan on high heat, add together the vegetable stock, pumpkin and onion powder.

2. Bring to a boil with constant stirring then reduce to medium-low heat. Allow to cook for 30 minutes, stirring occasionally.

3. Meanwhile, whip the heavy cream until it forms soft peaks. Place in the refrigerator.

4. Remove the soup from heat and blend until very smooth. Stir in the whipped cream, season to taste with salt and pepper then serve.

Nutrition Guide Per Serving:

Calories 209, Carbs 9.1g, Protein 5.4g, Fat 16.8g

Coconut Chicken Curry (Slow cooker)

Servings: 6

Prep Time: 10 minutes

Cook Time: 4 hours

Ingredients:

1 pound chicken, cut into bite size

2 tablespoons curry paste

1 onion, sliced thinly

1 2/3 cups coconut cream

14 ounces fresh spinach, chopped

Directions:

1. In the slow cooker, combine the chicken with curry paste, onion and coconut cream. Stir to combine.

2. Cover and cook for 4-5 hours on High or 6-8 hours on Low.

3. Stir in the spinach about 10 minutes before you serve and let heat through until spinach wilts.

Nutrition Guide Per Serving:

Calories 323, Carbs 7.4g, Protein 26g, Fat 20g

Zucchini And Herbs Soup (Stove top)

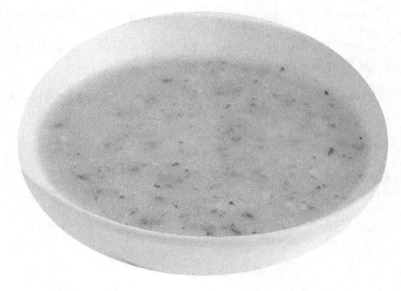

Servings: 4

Prep Time: 15 minutes

Cook Time: 20 minutes

Ingredients:

3 medium zucchini, cut into 1-inch pieces

3 cups low sodium chicken broth

1 teaspoon dried dill

Salt and freshly ground pepper, to taste

3/4 cup shredded reduced-fat Cheddar cheese

Directions:

1. In a medium saucepan on high heat, combine the zucchini with chicken broth and dill. Bring to a boil then reduce to a simmer.

2. Let cook, uncovered for 7 to 10 minutes, or until zucchini is tender.

3. Working in batches, transfer to a blender and blend until smooth. You could also use an immersion blender.

4. Return to the saucepan on medium-high. Stir in the cheese slowly until incorporated and melted. Season with salt and pepper and serve.

Nutrition Guide Per Serving:

Calories 109, Carbs 7g, Protein 10g, Fat 5.9g

Easy Celery Soup (Oven)

Servings: 4

Prep Time: 15 minutes

Cook Time: 25 minutes

Ingredients:

2 shallots, chopped roughly

4 cups sliced celery (1-inch pieces)

2 tablespoons extra-virgin olive oil

Salt and ground pepper, to taste

2 1/2 cups of reduced-sodium vegetable broth

Directions:

1. Preheat your oven to 450°F

2. In a large bowl, combine celery, shallots and olive oil. Season with salt and pepper and toss to mix well.

3. Spread out the mixture on a rimmed baking sheet. Roast for about 25 minutes, or until vegetables are tender. Stir once after the first 10 minutes.

4. Meanwhile, heat the broth in a saucepan.

5. Combine roasted vegetables with broth and puree until smooth.

Nutrition Guide Per Serving:

Calories 128, Carbs 10g, Protein 4g, Fat 8g

Chicken Endives Soup (Stove top)

Servings: 4

Prep Time: 5 minutes

Cook Time: 15 minutes

Ingredients:

1 (14-ounce) can fat-free, low-sodium chicken broth

1 (14.5-ounce) can stewed tomatoes, undrained, chopped

1 small head endives, chopped coarsely

1 cup cooked chicken breast, chopped

2 teaspoons olive oil

Directions:

1. In a large saucepan, mix together chicken broth and tomatoes. Bring to a boil on medium high heat then reduce the heat and let simmer for 5 minutes.

2. Stir in the endives, chicken and olive oil. Cook for additional 5 minutes.

Nutrition Guide Per Serving:

Calories 120, Carbs 7.8g, Protein 13.7g, Fat 4.5g

Easiest Onion Soup (Stove top)

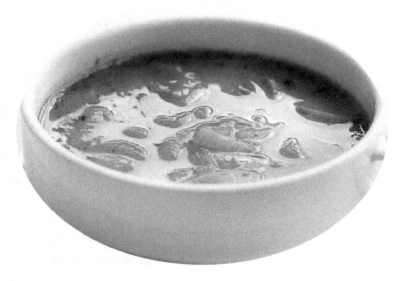

Servings: 6

Prep Time: 10 minutes

Cook Time: 45 minutes

Ingredients:

4 tablespoons ghee

4 large onions, sliced thinly

5 garlic cloves, chopped

4 cups chicken broth

Sea salt and black pepper, to taste

Directions:

1. Melt ghee in a large stockpot on medium heat. Add onions and cook until translucent.

2. Add the garlic and chicken broth then season to taste with salt and pepper.

3. Bring to a boil, then turn down the heat and let simmer for 30 to 40 minutes.

4. You can top with cheese when you serve.

Nutrition Guide Per Serving:

Calories 224, Carbs 9.3g, Protein 16.8g, Fat 11.8g

POULTRY MAIN DISH

Easiest Baked Chicken Breasts (Oven)
This helps you get dinner on the table very quickly.

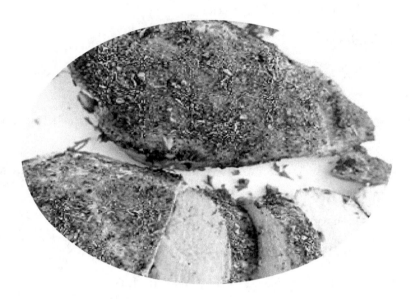

Servings: 4

Prep Time: 10 minutes

Cook Time: 30 minutes

Ingredients:

4 chicken breast halves, skinless, boneless

1/4 cup butter

1 teaspoon salt

Directions:

1. Preheat your oven to 350°F. Grease a baking dish lightly.

2. Add the butter to a saucepan on low heat and melt. Remove from heat and stir in the salt.

3. Place chicken in the baking dish and brush generously with the salted butter. Pour the remaining butter over.

4. Bake in the oven for 30 to 45 minutes, or until done to your preference.

Nutrition Guide Per Serving:

Calories 226, Carbs 0.2g, Protein 23.8g, Fat 14.3g

Rosemary Chicken And Bacon (Grill)
Everything comes together so perfectly.

Servings: 4

Prep Time: 10 minutes

Cook Time: 17 minutes

Ingredients:

4 chicken breast halves, skinless, boneless

4 thick bacon slices

Salt and pepper, to taste

4 teaspoons garlic powder

4 sprigs fresh rosemary

Directions:

1. Preheat your outdoor grill to medium-high heat and oil the grate lightly.

2. Sprinkle one chicken breast with garlic powder, salt and pepper. Place a sprig of rosemary on it then wrap with a slice of bacon. Use a toothpick to secure. Repeat with the remaining chicken breasts.

3. Place chicken on the grill and cook for 8 minutes per side, or until desired doneness.

Nutrition Guide Per Serving:

Calories 204, Carbs 2.2g, Protein 29.5g, Fat 8g

Creamy Ranch Chicken (Oven)

Servings: 8

Prep Time: 10 minutes

Cook Time: 45 minutes

Ingredients:

8 chicken breast halves, skinless, boneless

4 ounces pork rinds, crushed

1 envelope ranch salad dressing mix

3/4 cup grated Parmesan cheese

1/2 cup butter, melted

Directions:

1. Preheat your oven to 350°F. Spray a 9x13-inch baking dish with cooking spray.

2. In a bowl, mix together pork rinds, ranch dressing mix and Parmesan. Spread out the mixture in a thin layer on a flat dish.

3. Dip one chicken breast in butter then roll in the pork rind mixture until coated evenly. Place in the baking dish. Repeat with the rest of the chicken.

4. Bake in the oven for 45 minutes, or until desired doneness.

Nutrition Guide Per Serving:

Calories 347, Carbs 2.2g, Protein 34.2g, Fat 20.5g

Prosciutto Chicken Breast (Oven)

An excellent result with just three ingredients.

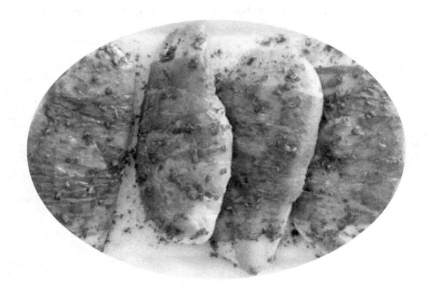

Servings: 4

Prep Time: 10 minutes

Cook Time: 25 minutes

Ingredients:

4 chicken breast halves, skinless, boneless

4 thin slices prosciutto

1/2 cup prepared basil pesto, divided

Directions:

1. Preheat your oven to 400°F and grease a sheet pan.

2. Spread 2 tablespoons of pesto on top of each chicken breast. Wrap each chicken breast with a slice of prosciutto. Arrange on the sheet pan.

3. Bake for 25 minutes, or until chicken is cooked through and prosciutto is crisped lightly.

Nutrition Guide Per Serving:

Calories 311, Carbs 2g, Protein 32g, Fat 19.5g

Easy Turkey Burgers (Grill)
A scrumptious meal for your family.

Servings: 4

Prep Time: 10 minutes

Cook Time: 20 minutes

Ingredients:

1 pound ground turkey

1/2 cup of water

1 packet of dry onion soup mix

Salt, to taste

Ground black pepper to taste

Directions:

1. Preheat your grill to high heat and oil the grate lightly.

2. Mix together ground turkey, water and onion soup mix in a large bowl. Add some salt and pepper (about 1/2 teaspoon each).

3. Mix with your hands and form into four patties.

5. Grill 7 to 10 minutes per side, or until cooked through.

Nutrition Guide Per Serving:

Calories 197, Carbs 6.4g, 23.4Protein g, Fat 8.4g

Chicken Breasts With Spinach Pesto (Oven)
A good way to eat more vegetables.

Servings: 4

Prep Time: 10 minutes

Cook Time: 45 minutes

Ingredients:

4 chicken breast halves, skinless, boneless

2 tablespoons basil pesto

1 1/2 cups fresh spinach, finely chopped

2 tablespoons grated Parmesan cheese

Directions:

1. Preheat your oven to 375°F.

2. In a bowl, mix together the pesto and spinach. Cover the bottom of a glass baking dish with half of the mixture.

3. Arrange the chicken breasts in the baking dish then pour the remaining pesto mixture over. Cover with aluminum foil.

4. Bake for 30 minutes. Remove the foil and sprinkle chicken with Parmesan cheese. Return to the oven then bake for 15 minutes more.

Nutrition Guide Per Serving:

Calories 180, Carbs 1.1g, Protein 26.4g, Fat 7.2g

Teriyaki Chicken (Grill)
Everyone in your home will love this.

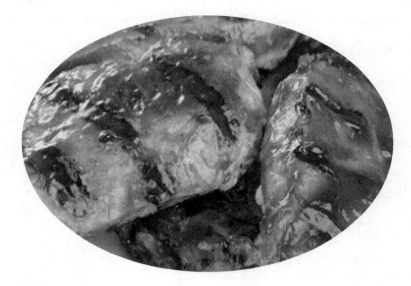

Servings: 4

Prep Time: 40 minutes

Cook Time: 20 minutes

Ingredients:

6 chicken breast halves, skinless, boneless

1 cup mayonnaise

3/4 cup soy sauce

Directions:

1. Mix mayonnaise and soy sauce together in a medium bowl. Add the chicken and toss to coat. Cover and set aside in the fridge for 30 minutes.

2. Preheat your outdoor grill to medium heat and oil the grate lightly.

3. Arrange the chicken on the grill, brush with some of the marinade and discard the remaining.

4. Cook until the chicken is done, about 10 minutes per side.

Nutrition Guide Per Serving:

Calories 612, Carbs 5.3g, Protein 44.5g, Fat 45.6g

Marinated Garlic Chicken (Grill)

Servings: 4

Prep Time: 10 minutes

Cook Time: 20 minutes

Ingredients:

4 chicken breasts skinless, boneless

4 garlic cloves, minced

1/2 cup soy sauce

Directions:

1. Combine minced garlic and soy sauce in a bowl. Add the chicken and toss to coat. Cover then set aside in the fridge for 1 hour.

2. Preheat your outdoor grill to medium high heat and oil the grate lightly.

3. Cook chicken on the grill until cooked through, about 10 to 15 minutes per side.

Nutrition Guide Per Serving:

Calories 154, Carbs 3.3g, Protein 27g, Fat 3g

Garlic Turkey Thighs (Slow cooker)
A simple but tasty combination.

Servings: 4

Prep Time: 20 minutes

Cook Time: 4 hours

Ingredients:

1 1/2 pounds turkey thighs, skinless, boneless

Lemon pepper, to taste

1 tablespoon olive oil

6 garlic cloves, minced

1 cup chicken broth

Directions:

1. Toss turkey breasts with lemon pepper.

55

2. Heat olive oil in a large skillet on medium-high heat. Add turkey and brown for about 10 minutes.

3. Combine turkey with the rest of the ingredients in the slow cooker. Cook for 4 hours on High.

Nutrition Guide Per Serving:

Calories 317, Carbs 8g, Protein 35g, Fat 14g

Juicy Pepper Chicken (Stove top)
Tasty, tangy and a little spicy.

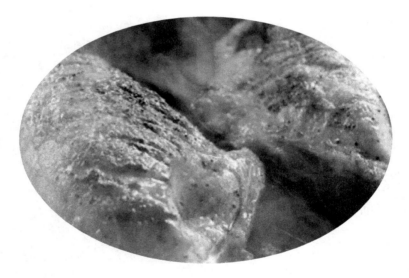

Servings: 2

Prep Time: 5 minutes

Cook Time: 15 minutes

Ingredients:

2 chicken breast halves, skinless, boneless

4 teaspoons butter

2 tablespoon ground black pepper, divided

2 tablespoons fresh lemon juice

Directions:

1. Melt butter in a skillet then stir in 1 tablespoon black pepper.

2. Add chicken to the skillet, drizzle with 1/2 of the lemon juice then sprinkle with the remaining 1 tablespoon pepper.

3. Cook for 7 minutes, flip over, drizzle with remaining lemon juice then cook until cooked through, about 5 to 7 minutes more.

Nutrition Guide Per Serving:

Calories 223, Carbs 5.6g, Protein 28g, Fat .79g

Cheesy Stuffed Chicken Breasts (Oven)
Once you eat this, it's going to become a favorite.

Servings: 4

Prep Time: 10 minutes

Cook Time: 25 minutes

Ingredients:

1 cup shredded mozzarella

1/2 cup grated cheddar cheese

1 tablespoon wholegrain mustard

4 skinless boneless chicken breast halves

8 smoked bacon slices

Directions:

1. Preheat your oven to 350°F. Mix the cheeses together with mustard in a bowl.

2. Using a sharp knife, cut a pocket into the side of each of the chicken breasts.

3. Stuff the cheese mixture into the pockets. Wrap each breast firmly with 2 slices of bacon. Season with salt and pepper.

4. Transfer to a baking sheet and bake for about 25 minutes, or until the chicken is cooked through.

Nutrition Guide Per Serving:

Calories 367, Carbs 0.2g, Protein 49g, Fat 19g

Marinated Grilled Chicken (Grill)

Servings: 4-6

Prep Time: 10 minutes

Cook Time: 30 minutes

Ingredients:

6 bone in, skin on chicken thighs

Juice from 4 lemons

2 tablespoons ground black pepper

2 tablespoons garlic salt

1/2 cup chopped fresh cilantro

Directions:

1. In a large ceramic bowl, whisk together lemon juice, black pepper, garlic salt and cilantro.

2. Add the chicken thighs and toss to coat. Cover and place in the refrigerator for at least 30 minutes.

3. Preheat your outdoor grill to medium heat and oil the grate lightly.

4. Place chicken on the grill and cook with occasional turning until cooked through, about 30 minutes.

Nutrition Guide Per Serving:

Calories 258, Carbs 4.4g, Protein 38g, Fat 10.1g

Slow Cooked Creamy Chicken (Slow cooker)

Servings: 4

Prep Time: 10 minutes

Cook Time: 6 hours

Ingredients:

3 skinless, boneless chicken thighs, cut bite size pieces

1/4 cup sour cream

1 (10.75 ounce) can cream of mushroom soup

1 (8 ounce) package of cream cheese

1 teaspoon Herbes de Provence

Directions:

1. In the slow cooker, mix together sour cream, mushroom soup, cream cheese and Herbes de Provence.

2. Add the chicken, cover and cook on Low for 6 hours.

Nutrition Guide Per Serving:

Calories 358, Carbs 7.6g, Protein 19.7g, Fat 27.6g

Chicken Garam Masala (Stove top)

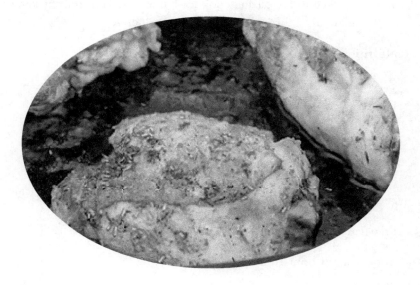

Servings: 4

Prep Time: 5 minutes

Cook Time: 15 minutes

Ingredients:

2 tablespoons butter

1 tablespoon olive oil

1 pound boneless, skinless chicken thighs, cut into bite size

3 tablespoons garam masala

Directions:

1. Heat butter and olive oil in a large skillet on medium high heat.

2. In a bowl, toss chicken pieces with garam masala.

3. Add chicken to the oil and cook for 5 minutes. Turn the chicken and cook until cooked through, about 7 to 10 minutes.

Nutrition Guide Per Serving:

Calories 241, Carbs 3.3g, Protein 25.7g, Fat 14g

Chicken Salsa Verde (Oven)

Servings: 4

Prep Time: 5 minutes

Cook Time: 1 hour 10 minutes

Ingredients:

6 chicken thighs, boneless skinless

1 cup Salsa Verde

1 onion, sliced thinly

2 garlic cloves, minced

Directions:

1. Preheat your oven to 350°F.

2. Place chicken thighs side by side in a glass baking dish. Top with the rest of the ingredients.

3. Cover and bake in the oven until chicken is cooked through, about 60 to 70 minutes.

4. Remove the chicken and use two forks to shred. Mix shredded chicken with cooking juices.

Nutrition Guide Per Serving:

Calories 254, Carbs 3.3g, Protein 22g, Fat 4g

Turkey Legs (Oven)
A very delicious turkey dinner.

Servings: 4

Prep Time: 10 minutes

Cook Time: 100 minutes

Ingredients:

3 bone-in turkey legs

1 teaspoon dried thyme

1 teaspoon poultry seasoning

1/2 cup butter, softened

1/2 cup water or chicken broth

Directions:

1. Preheat your oven to 350°F.

2. Rinse the turkey legs, pat dry with paper towels and place on a large roasting pan.

3. Use a sharp knife to cut a few long shallow pockets on both sides of the turkey.

4. In a small bowl, mix together the thyme, poultry seasoning, butter and some salt to taste. Rub the mixture all over the turkey, pressing into the cuts.

5. Pour 1/2 cup of water or broth into the roasting pan.

6. Roast for 1 hour 40 minutes, or until the turkey legs are cooked through.

7. Remove from the oven and let stand for 10 minute before serving.

Nutrition Guide Per Serving:

Calories 645, Carbs 1.7g, Protein 72g, Fat 37g

BEEF MAIN DISH

Good Time Rib Roast (Oven)
This is a meal to cook when you have a really special occasion.

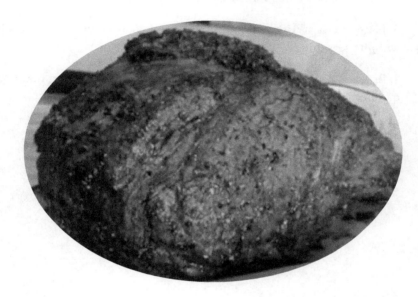

Servings: 6

Prep Time: 5 minutes

Cook Time: 1 hour 20 minutes

Ingredients:

1 beef rib roast (about 5 pounds)

1 teaspoon garlic powder

2 teaspoons salt

1 teaspoon of ground black pepper

Directions:

1. Make sure the roast is completely thawed then preheat your oven to 375°F.

2. In a small bowl, mix together garlic powder, salt and pepper.

3. Place the roast with fatty side up on a rack in a roasting pan. Rub all over with the seasoning.

4. Roast in the preheated oven for 1 hour 20 minutes. Let rest for about 10 minutes before cutting up.

Nutrition Guide Per Serving:

Calories 576, Carbs 0.6g, Protein 37g, Fat 46

Delightful Pot Roast (Slow cooker)
If you don't want to cook all day then this is for you.

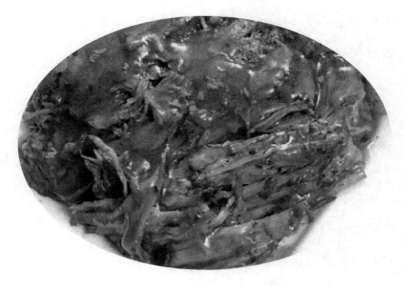

Servings: 12

Prep Time: 10 minutes

Cook Time: 4 hours

Ingredients:

5 1/2 pounds pot roast

1 1/4 cups water

1 package of dry onion soup mix

2 (10.75 ounce) cans of condensed cream of mushroom soup

Directions:

1. Add the water, onion soup mix and cream of mushroom soup to the slow cooker then mix together.

2. Add the roast to the pot and coat it with the mixture.

3. Cook for 3 to 4 hours on High or 8 to 9 hours on Low.

Nutrition Guide Per Serving:

Calories 426, Carbs 5g, Protein 45.7g, Fat 24g

Juicy Prime Rib Roast (Oven)
The marinade seeps into the meat to make it so delicious.

Servings: 15

Prep Time: 10 minutes

Cook Time: 1 hour 25 minutes

Ingredients:

1 prime rib roast (about 10 pounds)

2 tablespoons olive oil

2 teaspoons dried thyme

8 garlic cloves, minced

Salt and ground black pepper, to taste

Directions:

1. Preheat your oven to 500°F and place the roast fatty side up in a roasting pan.

2. Mix together the rest of the ingredients in a small bowl. Rub the mixture on the fatty side of the meat then set aside for 40 to 50 minutes.

3. Bake in the oven for 20 minutes. Reduce the temperature to 325°F and continue baking for additional 65 minutes.

4. Let rest for about 10 minutes before cutting up.

Nutrition Guide Per Serving:

Calories 562, Carbs 1g, Protein 30g, Fat 48g

Balsamic Filet Mignon (Stove top)
This is great with steamed vegetables.

Servings: 4

Prep Time: 5 minutes

Cook Time: 15 minutes

Ingredients:

4 (4 ounce) filet mignon steaks

Salt to taste

Freshly ground black pepper, to taste

1/2 cup dry red wine

1/2 cup balsamic vinegar

Directions:

1. Sprinkle each steak on both sides with salt and pepper.

2. Heat a skillet on medium-high heat. Add the steaks then cook until browned, about 1 minute per side.

3. Reduce to medium-low heat. Add the red wine and balsamic vinegar

4. Cover and let cook for 5 minutes. Flip to the other side and cook for additional 5 minutes.

5. Serve immediately with some of the glaze spooned over.

Nutrition Guide Per Serving:

Calories 368, Carbs 5.6g, Protein 20.5g, Fat 26.4g

Garlic Butter Sirloin Steak (Grill)

Melts in your mouth and it's simply wonderful!

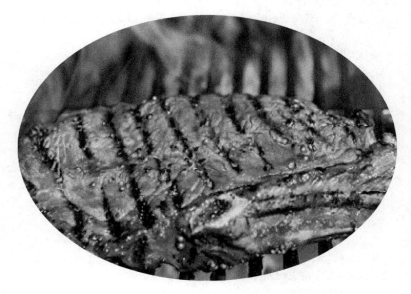

Servings: 8

Prep Time: 20 minutes

Cook Time: 10 minutes

Ingredients:

4 pounds of beef top sirloin steaks

1/2 cup butter

4 garlic cloves, minced

2 teaspoons garlic powder

Salt and pepper to taste

Directions:

1. Preheat your outdoor grill to high heat.

2. Melt the butter in a skillet on medium low heat. Stir in the minced garlic and garlic powder then let heat through. Set aside.

3. Salt and pepper each steak on both sides.

4. Grill steaks to desired doneness, about 4 to 5 minutes per side.

5. Transfer to plates and brush with the garlic butter generously. Let it sit for a few minutes before serving.

Nutrition Guide Per Serving:

Calories 453, Carbs 1g, Protein 38g, Fat 32.4g

Creamy Beef On Toast (Stove top)

This is nice comfort food that you can enjoy with toast.

Servings: 4

Prep Time: 10 minutes

Cook Time: 10 minutes

Ingredients:

1 (8 ounce) jar dried beef

2 tablespoons almond flour

2 tablespoons butter

1 1/2 cups warm milk

1 pinch of cayenne pepper

Directions:

1. Melt butter on low heat in a medium saucepan. Whisk in the almond flour to make a roux.

2. Gradually stir in the milk. Increase to medium-high and cook with constant stirring until thickened.

3. Stir in the beef and the cayenne pepper. Allow to heat through then serve on your favorite keto bread toast.

Nutrition Guide Per Serving:

Calories 197, Carbs 7g, Protein 21g, Fat 8.7g

Family Beef Tenderloin
A delightful dish for family dinners.

Servings: 6

Prep Time: 5 minutes

Cook Time: 45 minutes

Ingredients:

1 (3 pound) beef tenderloin roast

3/4 cup soy sauce

1/2 cup melted butter

Directions:

1. Preheat your oven to 350°F. Melt butter on low heat in a saucepan and set aside.

2. Add roast to a shallow glass baking dish. Pour in the melted butter and soy sauce.

3. Bake for 15 minutes in the oven, flip over then continue baking for 30 to 35 minutes. Baste with the juices occasionally.

4. Let it sit for at least 10 minutes before cutting up.

Nutrition Guide Per Serving:

Calories 590, Carbs 2.5g, Protein 59g, Fat 33.1g

Tender Beef Roast (Slow cooker)

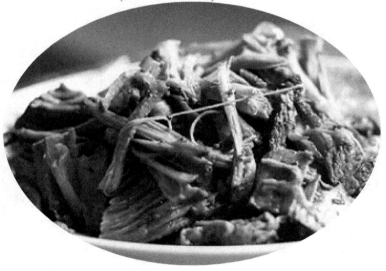

Servings: 6

Prep Time: 5 minutes

Cook Time: 8 hours

Ingredients:

3 pounds of rump roast

1 can condensed beef broth (10.5 ounce)

1 can condensed cream of mushroom soup (10.75 ounce)

Directions:

1. Simply dump everything in the slow cooker.

2. Cook for 8 hours on Low.

Nutrition Guide Per Serving:

Calories 308, Carbs 3.4g, Protein 35.2g, Fat 16.2g

Everyday Roast Beef

A basic recipe you can make anytime.

Servings: 6

Prep Time: 5 minutes

Cook Time: 1 hour

Ingredients:

3 pounds beef eye of round roast

1/4 teaspoon freshly ground black pepper

1/2 teaspoon kosher salt

1/2 teaspoon garlic powder

Directions:

1. Preheat your oven to 375°F. Using cotton twine, tie the roast at 3 inch intervals.

2. Place in a roasting pan then season with the salt, pepper and garlic powder.

3. Bake for 60 minutes in the oven. Remove from the oven and keep warm for 10 to 15 minutes before cutting up.

Nutrition Guide Per Serving:

Calories 484, Carbs 0.3g, Protein 44.6g, Fat 32.3g

Salty Prime Rib Roast (Oven)
This is juicy and incredibly flavored by kosher salt.

Servings: 6

Prep Time: 10 minutes

Cook Time: 4 hours 30 minutes

Ingredients:

4 pounds prime rib roast

2 cups coarse kosher salt

1 tablespoon seasoning salt

1 tablespoon ground black pepper

Directions:

1. Preheat your oven to 210°F

2. Spread a layer of kosher salt over the bottom of a roasting pan. Place the roast on the pan with the bone side down.

3. Sprinkle with seasoning salt and pepper. Cover the meat with a layer of kosher salt.

4. Roast in the oven for 4 hours 30 minutes, or until cooked through.

5. Transfer to a platter and let rest for 30 minutes. Scrape off all the kosher salt before cutting up.

Nutrition Guide Per Serving:

Calories 391, Carbs 1.1g, Protein 36g, Fat 26g

Grilled Hamburgers (Grill)
You can serve this on lettuce or keto buns with your favorite toppings.

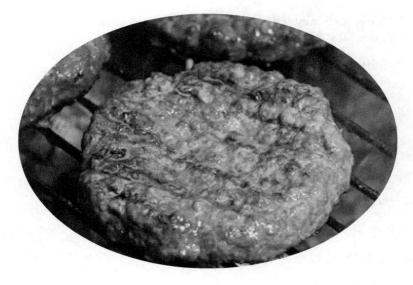

Servings: 4

Prep Time: 5 minutes

Cook Time: 10 minutes

Ingredients:

1 pound of ground beef

1 egg

Steak sauce, to taste

2 garlic cloves, minced

Directions:

1. Preheat your outdoor grill to high heat.

2. Mix the ground beef with egg and garlic in a medium bowl. Mix in the steak sauce until you have a sticky mixture (usually about 1 tablespoon).

3. Form into 4 balls then press down to make patties.

4. Grill for 5 minutes on one side then flip and grill on the other side for additional 5 minutes, or until done.

Nutrition Guide Per Serving:

Calories 374, Carbs 1.1g, Protein 21g, Fat 31.3g

BBQ Beef Brisket (Oven)

Servings: 8

Prep Time: 10 minutes

Cook Time: 4 hours

Ingredients:

4 pounds beef brisket

1 teaspoon garlic powder

Salt and freshly ground black pepper, to taste

1 cup water

1 cup barbecue sauce

Directions:

1. Preheat your oven to 325°F.

2. Place brisket in a roasting pan then sprinkle on both sides with salt, pepper and garlic powder.

3. Cover and roast for 3 hours.

4. After 3 hours, remove from the oven and slice. Return to the pan then add water and barbecue sauce. Let the mixture cover the meat. Cook for additional 1 hour.

Nutrition Guide Per Serving:

Calories 650, Carbs 9.8g, Protein 34.1g, Fat 53.3g

Easiest Cube Steaks

Servings: 4

Prep Time: 15 minutes

Cook Time: 1 hour

Ingredients:

4 cube steaks (1/2 pound each)

1 (10.5 ounce) can of condensed French onion soup

Directions:

1. Preheat your oven to 350°F

2. Brown the cube steaks on both sides in a large skillet on medium heat.

3. In a 13x9 inch baking dish, place the meat in a single layer then pour the onion soup on top.

4. Bake for 1 hour.

Nutrition Guide Per Serving:

Calories 433, Carbs 6.5g, Protein 50g, Fat 22.4g

Poblano Pot Roast (Slow cooker)

Servings: 6

Prep Time: 10 minutes

Cook Time: 8 hours

Ingredients:

4 pounds beef chuck roast

5 poblano peppers

1/4 cup of butter

1 packet of dry au jus mix

1 packet of ranch dressing mix

Directions:

1. Add the roast to the slow cooker. Press down at the middle of the roast and place the peppers, butter and seasonings.

2. Cook for 8 hours on Low.

Nutrition Guide Per Serving:

Calories 533, Carbs 5.7g, Protein 36.4g, Fat 39.3g

Spicy Burgers (Grill)

Serve these moist and flavorful burgers on your favorite keto buns.

Servings: 4

Prep Time: 15 minutes

Cook Time: 10 minutes

Ingredients:

1 pound ground beef

1 teaspoon of beef bouillon granules

1 (4 ounce) can of diced green chilies, drained

4 slices of Monterey Jack cheese

Directions:

1. Preheat your outdoor grill to high heat and oil the grate lightly.

2. Mix together the ground beef, bouillon and green chilies in a medium bowl. Form into 4 patties.

3. Grill for 5 minutes on each side, or until cooked through.

4. About 2 minutes to the end of cooking time, place a slice of cheese on each patty.

Nutrition Guide Per Serving:

Calories 340, Carbs 1.7g, Protein 25.8g, Fat 24.8g

Spinach Meatloaf (Oven)

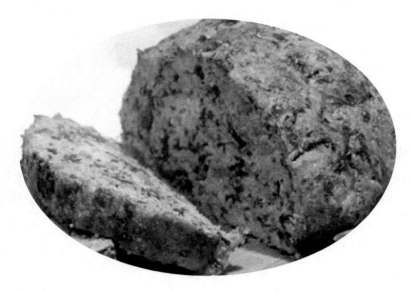

Servings: 4

Prep Time: 5 minutes

Cook Time: 30 minutes

Ingredients:

1 pound ground beef

12 ounces ground pork sausage

1 (13.5 ounces) can spinach, drained.

1 teaspoon garlic and onion spice blend

Salt and pepper, to taste

Directions:

1. Mix everything together, shape then place in an oven safe dish.

2. Bake at 350°F for 30 minutes, or until cooked through.

Nutrition Guide Per Serving:

Calories 470, Carbs 3g, Protein 34.4g, Fat 21.4g

PORK MAIN DISH

Parmesan Pork Chops (Oven)
Simply scrumptious.

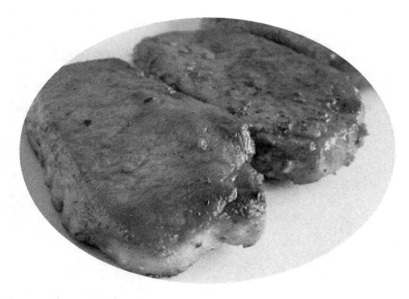

Servings: 4

Prep Time: 10 minutes

Cook Time: 35 minutes

Ingredients:

4 boneless pork chops, trimmed

2 eggs

2 teaspoons Cajun seasoning

1/2 cup grated Parmesan cheese

Directions:

1. Preheat your oven to 350°F. Spray cooking spray on a baking dish.

2. Break the eggs into a shallow bowl and whisk together. In a plate, mix together the Cajun seasoning and Parmesan cheese.

3. Working one at a time, dip pork chop into the egg then roll in the Cajun seasoning mixture until fully coated. Transfer to the greased baking dish.

4. Bake for 35 to 40 minutes, or until golden.

Nutrition Guide Per Serving:

Calories 247, Carbs 1.2g, Protein 31g, Fat 12.7g

Ham And Leeks (Oven)

Servings: 4

Prep Time: 5 minutes

Cook Time: 20 minutes

Ingredients:

8 small leeks, white part only

8 slices of cooked ham

6 tablespoons sour cream

2 tablespoons Dijon mustard

1 cup cheddar cheese, grated

Directions:

1. Preheat your oven to 350°F.

2. Boil salted water in a pan, add the leeks and cook for 4 to 5 minutes. Drain, cool under a running tap and pat dry with paper towels.

3. In a bowl, mix together the sour cream, mustard and cheddar cheese. Season to taste with salt and pepper.

4. Wrap each leek with a slice of cooked ham. Arrange in one layer on a baking sheet. Top with the cheese mixture.

5. Bake for 15 to 20 minutes, or until golden brown and bubbly. Serve with keto buns.

Nutrition Guide Per Serving:

Calories 295, Carbs 6g, Protein 20g, Fat 21g

Quick Pork Chops (Stove top)

Servings: 4

Prep Time: 10 minutes

Cook Time: 16 minutes

Ingredients:

4 (7-ounce) bone-in pork loin chops

3 garlic cloves, minced

3 tablespoons soy sauce

6 tablespoons apple cider vinegar, divided

1-1/2 teaspoons arrowroot powder

Directions:

1. Add pork chops to a large skillet on medium heat. Brown for 2 minutes per side.

2. Mix the garlic and soy sauce with 5 tablespoons of vinegar. Pour the mixture over the pork.

3. Bring to a boil then reduce the heat, cover and let simmer for 8 to 10 minutes.

4. Mix the reserved vinegar with arrowroot powder then stir into the skillet. Cook and stir for about 1 minute then remove from heat.

Nutrition Guide Per Serving:

Calories 224, Carbs 2g, Protein 32g, Fat 8g

Spicy Pork Tenderloin (Oven, Stove top)
Serve this lovely dinner over a bed of salad.

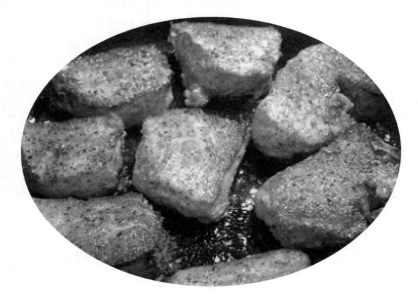

Servings: 6

Prep Time: 10 minutes

Cook Time: 25 minutes

Ingredients:

2 (12-14-ounce) pork tenderloins, fat trimmed

Olive oil cooking spray

2 teaspoons 5-spice powder, divided

1 cup cherry tomatoes, cut in half

1 large red onion

Directions:

1. Preheat your oven to 450°F. Line a baking sheet with aluminum foil then spray lightly with cooking spray.

2. Season pork tenderloins with 1 teaspoon of 5-spice powder then place in the baking sheet. Bake until cooked through, about20-30 minutes.

3. Meanwhile, spray cooking spray on a skillet on medium heat. Add the onion and cook until just softened. Add the cherry tomatoes and continue cooking until tomatoes soften and onions are very tender.

4. Slice the pork tenderloins and serve with onion/tomato mixture.

Nutrition Guide Per Serving:

Calories 239, Carbs 6.2g, Protein 32g, Fat 9.3g

Stir Fry Pork Chops (Stove top)

Servings: 4

Prep Time: 5 minutes

Cook Time: 20 minutes

Ingredients:

4 bone-in pork chops, about 1 inch thick

1/4 cup almond flour

1/2 teaspoon pepper

2 teaspoons seasoned salt

2 tablespoons butter

Directions:

1. Add the flour to a shallow dish. Rub pork chops all over with pepper and seasoned salt.

2. Dredge in the flour and shake off excess flour.

3. Add butter to a large skillet on medium-high heat. When butter melts, add the pork chops and cook for about 7-10 minutes on each side, or until done to your liking. You may have to work in batches if you have large pork chops.

4. Transfer to a plate and let cool for at least 5 minutes before serving.

Nutrition Guide Per Serving:

Calories 475, Carbs 4.5g, Protein 49.4g, Fat 26.3g

Glazed Pulled Pork (Slow cooker)
Pulled pork with a smoky barbecue flavor.

Servings: 12 - 15

Prep Time: 5 minutes

Cook Time: 8 hours

Ingredients:

5 pound pork butt roast

2 tablespoons Cajun seasoning

1/4 cup Truvia brown sugar blend

1 tablespoon liquid smoke

1/4 cup apple cider vinegar

Directions:

1. In a large slow cooker, combine liquid smoke and vinegar with 1/4 cup of water.

2. Mix together Cajun seasoning and brown sugar blend. Rub the mixture all over the pork roast and pour the rest into the slow cooker. Add the pork roast to the slow cooker.

3. Cover and cook on Low for 12 hours or on High for 7-8 hours.

4. Remove from the slow cooker and shred with two forks. Serve shredded pork with cooking juices.

Nutrition Guide Per Serving:

Calories 540, Carbs 1.8g, Protein 66g, Fat 22.3g

Almond Flour Coated Pork Chops (Stove top)

Another easy way to get pork chops on the table very quickly.

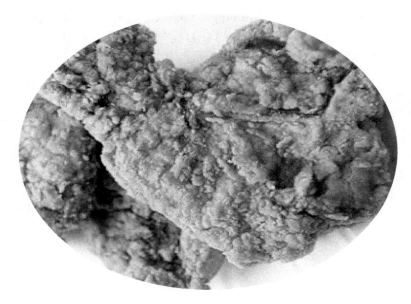

Servings: 4

Prep Time: 10 minutes

Cook Time: 20 minutes

Ingredients:

4 pork chops

1 cup vegetable oil

1/2 cup almond flour

Seasoning salt, to taste

Salt and pepper, to taste

Directions:

1. In a large skillet, heat the oil on medium heat.

2. In a plastic bag, combine almond flour with seasoning salt, salt and pepper. Add the pork chops then shake to coat with the mixture.

3. Remove pork chops from the bag, shake off excess and add to the hot oil. Cook for about 5 to 6 minutes per side, or until cooked through.

Nutrition Guide Per Serving:

Calories 304, Carbs 2g, Protein 26g, Fat 27g

Cheesy Skillet Pork Chops (Stove top)
A very easy way to cook mouthwatering pork chops.

Servings: 4

Prep Time: 10 minutes

Cook Time: 20 minutes

Ingredients:

4 pork chops

2 tablespoons of olive oil

1 cup of fresh lemon juice

1/2 cup of crumbled feta cheese with basil and tomatoes

1 tablespoon Italian seasoning

Directions:

1. Heat the oil in a large skillet on medium heat.

2. Dip the pork chops in the lemon juice then sprinkle all over with Italian seasoning

3. Add pork chops to the hot oil and cook for 5-6 minutes on both sides.

4. Turn the heat down to low, add the feta cheese and cook for 5 minutes more.

Nutrition Guide Per Serving:

Calories 318, Carbs 6.5g, Protein 25.7g, Fat 21.6g

Teriyaki Pork Kebabs (Grill)

Servings: 4

Prep Time: 15 minutes

Cook Time: 14 minutes

Ingredients:

4 pound pork tenderloin, cut into 1 inch cubes

1 tablespoon red wine vinegar

2 tablespoons teriyaki sauce

1/2 teaspoon red pepper flakes

1 tablespoon vegetable oil

Directions:

1. Preheat your outdoor grill to medium heat and oil the grate lightly.

2. In a large bowl, mix together red wine vinegar, teriyaki sauce, red pepper flakes and vegetable oil. Add the pork cubes then toss to coat.

3. Arrange the pork cubes on skewers and reserve the remaining mixture.

4. Cook for 12 to 14 minutes, turning frequently and basting with the reserved teriyaki mixture as required.

Nutrition Guide Per Serving:

Calories 155, Carbs 3g, Protein 19g, Fat 78g

Chorizo Made At Home
A spicy sausage you can simply crumble and fry whenever you want.

Servings:

Prep Time: 15 minutes

Cook Time: minutes

Ingredients:

2 1/2 pounds ground pork or ground beef

1/2 cup crushed red pepper flakes

3 teaspoons dried oregano

1 garlic clove

1/2 cup white vinegar

Directions:

1. Pour 1/2 cup of water into a blender then add red pepper flakes, oregano, garlic and vinegar. Process until smooth.

2. Add the ground pork to a bowl then top with the blended mixture. Cover and place in the fridge for 8 to 10 hours.

3. Pour off any accumulated water then refrigerate to use later.

Nutrition Guide Per Serving:

Calories 321, Carbs 5.4g, Protein 26.2g, Fat 22g

Spicy Sausage Patties (Stove top)

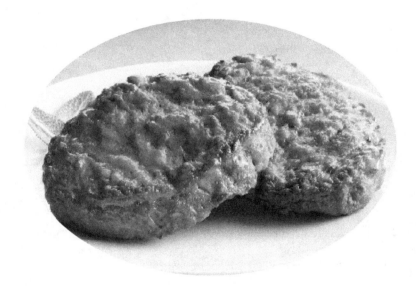

Servings: 4

Prep Time: 10 minutes

Cook Time: 15 minutes

Ingredients:

1 pound fresh, ground pork sausage

1 1/2 tablespoons ground cumin

1 tablespoon crushed red pepper

2 garlic cloves, minced

Salt to taste

Directions:

1. Combine all the ingredients together in a bowl. Use your hands to form into patties.

2. Spray a skillet with cooking spray and place on medium heat. Fry patties until done on both sides.

Nutrition Guide Per Serving:

Calories 490, Carbs 4.3g, Protein 14.5g, Fat 46g

Omelet With Ground Pork (Stove top)
Taste real good and you can eat it anytime of the day.

Servings: 2

Prep Time: 5 minutes

Cook Time: 5 minutes

Ingredients:

3 eggs

6 ounces ground pork

1 pinch pepper

2 1/2 tablespoons Worcestershire sauce

2 tablespoons vegetable oil

Directions:

1. Whisk the eggs in a medium bowl then whisk in ground pork, pepper and Worcestershire sauce.

2. Add oil to a skillet and heat on medium heat. Fry until golden on both sides.

Nutrition Guide Per Serving:

Calories 407, Carbs 1.6g, Protein 25.8g, Fat 33.6g

SEAFOOD MAIN DISH

Cajun Grilled Shrimp (Grill)

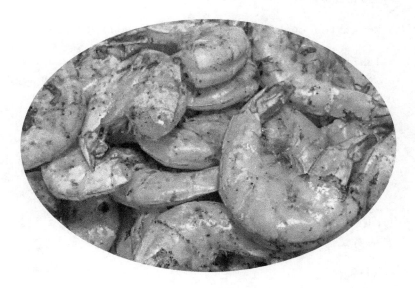

Servings: 8

Prep Time: 5 minutes

Cook Time: 5 minutes

Ingredients:

1 pound medium shrimp, peeled, deveined

1 lime, juiced

3 tablespoons Cajun seasoning

1 tablespoon vegetable oil

Directions:

1. In a medium bowl, mix together lime juice, Cajun seasoning and oil.

2. Add the shrimp and toss until completely coated. Cover and refrigerate for 20 minutes.

3. Preheat your outdoor grill to medium heat and oil the grate lightly.

4. Take shrimp out of the marinade then shake off excess marinade. Cook on the grill for about 2 minutes per side. The shrimp should no longer be transparent in the center and should be bright pink outside.

Nutrition Guide Per Serving:

Calories 70, Carbs 2.4g, Protein 9.7g, Fat 2.5g

Quick Tomato Salmon (Oven)
This elegant dish goes well with sautéed vegetables.

Servings: 4

Prep Time: 10 minutes

Cook Time: 20 minutes

Ingredients:

4 (6 ounce) boneless salmon fillets

2 tablespoons dried basil

2 tomatoes, sliced thinly

2 tablespoons olive oil

4 tablespoons grated Parmesan cheese

Directions:

1. Preheat your oven to 375°F. Place a piece of aluminum foil on a baking sheet then spray it with cooking spray.

2. Arrange the fish on the foil, sprinkle with the basil and arrange tomato slices on top. Sprinkle with Parmesan cheese then drizzle with olive oil.

3. Bake in the oven for about 20 minutes, or until the salmon is cooked through.

Nutrition Guide Per Serving:

Calories 404, Carbs 4g, Protein 35.9g, Fat 26.7g

Weeknight Trout (Oven)

Servings: 4

Prep Time: 15 minutes

Cook Time: 10 minutes

Ingredients:

1/2 cup butter

4 (8 ounce) whole trout, butterflied, deboned

Salt and freshly ground black pepper, to taste

Juice of 2 lemons

4 tablespoons fresh flat-leaf parsley, chopped

Directions:

1. Melt the butter in a saucepan.

2. Preheat your oven broiler to high heat. Place aluminum foil in a baking sheet.

3. Place trout on the foil with skin side down. Drizzle each fish with some melted butter (about 1 teaspoon each). Season liberally with salt and pepper.

4. Place the baking sheet in the oven about 5 or 6 inches below the heat source. Broil for 2 or 3 minutes, or until fish is firm and opaque. Remove from the oven.

5. Add lemon juice and parsley to the remaining butter in the saucepan. Bring to a boil on high heat, with constant stirring.

6. Serve fish with the butter sauce poured on top.

Nutrition Guide Per Serving:

Calories 466, Carbs 1.5g, Protein 39.7g, Fat 33.3g

Cheesy Salmon (Oven)

Put this together for a quick weeknight meal with a green salad.

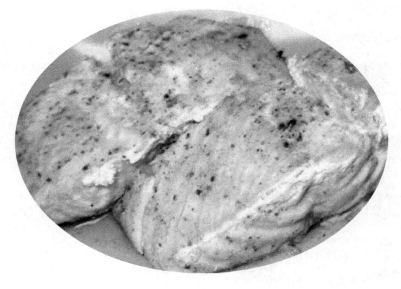

Servings: 4

Prep Time: 10 minutes

Cook Time: 20 minutes

Ingredients:

4 (6 ounce) salmon fillets

4 tablespoons butter, softened

1/2 cup grated sharp cheddar cheese

4 tablespoons chopped fresh parsley

4 tablespoons slivered almond

Directions:

1. Preheat your oven to 350°F. Rub butter liberally on the bottom of a large baking sheet.

2. Place the fish fillets side by side on the baking sheet then season with salt and pepper.

3. Mix the cheddar cheese, parsley and almond together in a bowl. Scoop the mixture on top of the fish, patting down gently.

4. Bake until the salmon is cooked through and the top is crispy and golden, about 17 to 20 minutes.

Nutrition Guide Per Serving:

Calories 522, Carbs 1.2g, Protein 41g, Fat 39g

Cheesy Grilled Cod (Grill)
A nutrient-packed meal for everyone.

Servings: 4

Prep Time: 15 minutes

Cook Time: 8 minutes

Ingredients:

4 skinless cod fillets

4 thin slices of ham

2 scallions, sliced

1/2 cup grated cheddar

Oil

Directions:

1. Preheat your outdoor grill to high heat. Grease a large shallow, heatproof dish lightly.

2. Place the fillets side by side in the dish then brush with a little oil. Cook for 3 minutes.

3. Meanwhile, mix together the scallions and cheese.

4. Remove the dish from the grill and flip over the fish. Top each fillet with a slice of ham and also the cheese mixture. Sprinkle with salt and pepper.

5. Return the dish to the grill and cook until the fish flakes easily with a fork, about 5 minutes.

Nutrition Guide Per Serving:

Calories , Carbs g, Protein g, Fat g

Oven Fried Shrimp (Oven)

Servings: 4

Prep Time: 5 minutes

Cook Time: 10 minutes

Ingredients:

1 pound large shrimp, cooked

1 1/2 ounces pork rinds, crushed

6 tablespoons grated Parmesan cheese

Directions:

1. Preheat your oven to 400°F

2. In a large bowl, mix the crushed pork rinds with parmesan. Add the shrimp and toss to coat.

3. Bake for 10 minutes.

Nutrition Guide Per Serving:

Calories 337, Carbs 1.0g, Protein 46g, Fat 16g

Greek Style Tilapia (Oven)

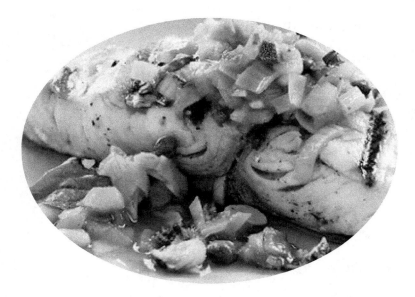

Servings: 6

Prep Time: 5 minutes

Cook Time: 20 minutes

Ingredients:

6 (6-ounce) tilapia fillets

1/2 cup sliced ripe olives

1/2 cup water-packed artichoke hearts, chopped

1 cup canned Italian diced tomatoes

1/2 cup crumbled feta cheese

Directions:

1. Preheat your oven to 400°F. Coat a large baking sheet with cooking spray.

2. Arrange the fillets on the baking sheet then top with olives, artichoke hearts, tomatoes and cheese.

3. Bake until the fish easily flakes with a fork, about 15-20 minutes.

Nutrition Guide Per Serving:

Calories 197, Carbs 5g, Protein 34g, Fat 4g

Easy Baked Halibut (Oven)
Curried halibut bursting with wonderful flavor.

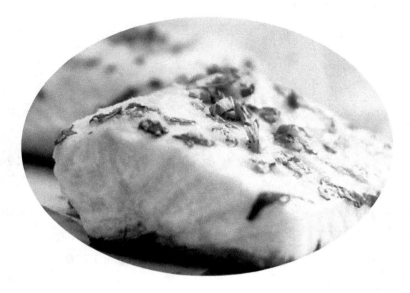

Servings: 4

Prep Time: 15 minutes

Cook Time: 25 minutes

Ingredients:

4 (6 ounce) Halibut fillets

1 teaspoon curry paste

1 cup sour cream

Directions:

1. Preheat your oven to 325°F. Spray cooking spray on a baking sheet.

2. Mix curry paste and sour cream together in a bowl.

3. Spread the fish fillets on one side with the mixture. Place on the baking sheet with the coated side down then spread the remaining mixture on top.

4. Bake until the halibut easily flakes with a fork, about 25 minutes.

Nutrition Guide Per Serving:

Calories 393, Carbs 2.7g, Protein 31g, Fat 28g

Lemon Pepper Rosemary Cod (Oven)

Servings: 4

Prep Time: 5 minutes

Cook Time: 7 minutes

Ingredients:

4 cod fillets

1/2 cup butter, cut into pieces

1 small bunch rosemary

3 tablespoons fresh lemon juice

Lemon pepper, to taste

Directions:

1. Preheat your oven to 350°F. Place the fish in an oven-safe dish.

2. Dot the fish with butter, sprinkle with rosemary leaves and lemon pepper then drizzle with the lemon juice.

3. Cook in the oven for 7 minutes, or until cooked through.

Nutrition Guide Per Serving:

Calories 305, Carbs 1g, Protein 21.8g, Fat 24.1g

Easy Baked Halibut (Oven)
You can't have enough of this delightful meal.

Servings: 4

Prep Time: 5 minutes

Cook Time: 10 minutes

Ingredients:

4 fresh halibut fillets

2 tablespoons packed fresh basil leaves, chopped roughly

1/4 cup butter

Seasoning salt, to taste

3 tablespoons almond meal

Directions:

1. Preheat your oven to 400°F. Place parchment paper on a large rimmed baking sheet.

2. Arrange the fillets on the parchment paper.

3. Combine butter and basil leaves in a food processor and process until smooth. Spread about half of the basil butter on the halibut fillets and refrigerate the rest.

4. Sprinkle seasoning salt on the fish then sprinkle with almond meal.

5. Bake for about 10 minutes, or until the fish is flaky and the tops are light brown and crispy.

6. Serve warm, topped with the basil butter.

Nutrition Guide Per Serving:

Calories 394, Carbs 1.3g, Protein 60g, Fat 14g

SIDE DISH

Mushroom Soup (Stove top)
Makes a warm side dish to a meaty dinner.

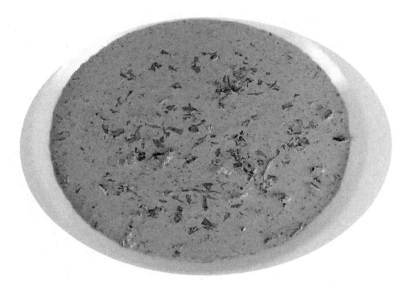

Servings: 4

Prep Time: 8 minutes

Cook Time: 5 minutes

Ingredients:

1 pound mushrooms, cleaned, sliced

1 cup water

1/4 cup heavy cream

1 tablespoon olive oil

1/4 cup of grated parmesan cheese

Directions:

1. Add 1 cup of water to a saucepan and bring to a boil. Add the mushrooms and cook on medium heat for 5 minutes.

2. Drain then transfer mushrooms to a blender. Puree and gradually add the heavy cream and olive oil.

3. Pour into a bowl and stir in the cheese. Season to taste with a little pepper if you like.

Nutrition Guide Per Serving:

Calories 207, Carbs 3g, Protein 9.7g, Fat 18g

Crispy Kale Chips (Oven)
Everyone will ask for more of these.

Servings: 6

Prep Time: 10 minutes

Cook Time: 10 minutes

Ingredients:

1 bunch of kale

1 teaspoon seasoned salt

1 tablespoon olive oil

Directions:

1. Preheat your oven to 350°F. Place parchment paper on a cookie sheet.

2. Wash and dry the kale then cut the leaves into bite size.

3. Place kale on the cookie sheet, drizzle with olive oil then sprinkle with the seasoning salt.

4. Bake for 12 to 15 minutes, or until the edges start to turn brown.

Nutrition Guide Per Serving:

Calories 58, Carbs 7.7g, Protein 2.6g, Fat 2.7g

Sautéed Bok Choy (Stove Top)
A quick and easy side to any meaty dish.

Servings: 2

Prep Time: 5 minutes

Cook Time: 5 minutes

Ingredients:

5 heads baby bok choy, trimmed, leaves separated

1 tablespoon olive oil

1/2 teaspoon ground cinnamon

1 garlic clove, minced

2 tablespoons water

Directions:

1. In a large skillet, heat the oil on medium-high heat. Add the ginger and cinnamon then cook with constant stirring for just 30 seconds.

2. Add the bok choy and 2 tablespoons of water. Stir then cover and cook for about 2 minutes, or until the bok choy is wilted.

Nutrition Guide Per Serving:

Calories 94, Carbs 6g, Protein 4g, Fat 7.2g

Lemon Cauliflower "Rice" (Microwave)
A flavorful side dish any time.

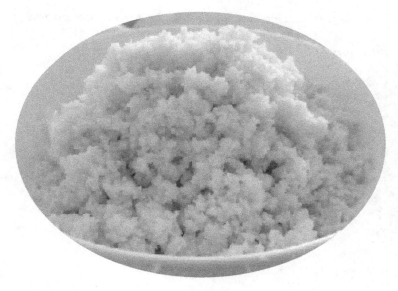

Servings: 4

Prep Time: 15 minutes

Cook Time: 10 minutes

Ingredients:

1 head cauliflower, broken into florets

1 tablespoon water

1 lemon, juiced and zested

Directions:

1. Add cauliflower florets to a food processor. Process until it becomes grainy like rice.

2. Transfer to a microwave-safe dish. Add 1 tablespoon of water, cover and microwave on high for about 7 minutes.

3. Remove from microwave and stir in the lemon juice and zest.

Nutrition Guide Per Serving:

Calories 92, Carbs 9.7g, Protein 3.2g, Fat 6g

Roasted Cabbage (Oven)

Sweet roasted cabbage with a nutty flavor.

Servings: 6

Prep Time: 10 minutes

Cook Time: 30 minutes

Ingredients:

1/2 head cabbage, cut into 4 wedges

2 tablespoon extra-virgin olive oil

Kosher salt, to taste

Freshly ground black pepper, to taste

Directions:

1. Preheat your oven to 450°F and place the rack at the middle position. Place foil on a rimmed sheet pan.

2. Place the cabbage wedges on the sheet pan side by side. Drizzle with half of the olive oil then season with salt and pepper. Flip over then season and drizzle with oil again.

3. Roast in the oven for about 15 minutes, flip over and roast for additional 15 minutes, or until deeply browned and tender.

Nutrition Guide Per Serving:

Calories 96, Carbs 8.8g, Protein 2g, Fat 6.8g

Keto Mashed Cauliflower (Stove top)

A good alternative to mashed potatoes.

Servings: 4

Prep Time: 10 minutes

Cook Time: 10 minutes

Ingredients:

1 medium head cauliflower, cut into florets

2 garlic cloves, minced

1/2 cup whipped cream cheese

1 tablespoon butter

Seasoned salt, to taste

Directions:

1. Add water and a little salt to a large pot and bring to a boil. Add the cauliflower and cook for about 6 minutes, or until tender.

2. Drain and use paper towels to pat dry.

3. Combine with the rest of the ingredients in a food processor. Process to mashed potato consistency.

Nutrition Guide Per Serving:

Calories 67, Carbs 9g, Protein 4g, Fat 5.5g

Roasted Broccoli (Oven)

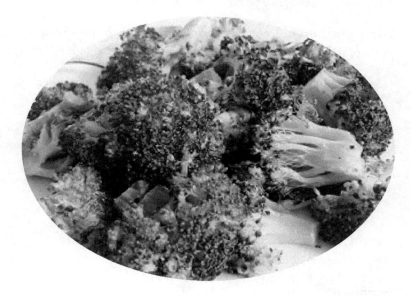

Servings: 4

Prep Time: 10 minutes

Cook Time: 20 minutes

Ingredients:

1 large bunch of broccoli (about 14 ounces)

1 tablespoon olive oil

Salt and ground black pepper, to taste

1 teaspoon garlic powder

Lemon juice

Directions:

1. Preheat your oven to 400°F.

2. Cut the broccoli into florets, peel and slice the stalk.

3. In a bowl, toss broccoli pieces with olive oil then spread out on a sheet pan. Sprinkle with garlic powder then season to taste with salt and pepper.

4. Roast in the oven for about 18 to 20 minutes, or until tender.

5. Serve, drizzled with lemon juice.

Nutrition Guide Per Serving:

Calories 64, Carbs 6.5g, Protein 2.9g, Fat 3.8g

Easy Cucumber Salad
A fresh salad side dish for grilled chicken or beef.

Servings: 6

Prep Time: 15 minutes

Cook Time: minutes

Ingredients:

1 large English cucumber, sliced

1 medium red onion, sliced thinly

2 cups cherry tomatoes, halved

1/2 red wine vinegar

3/4 cup crumbled feta cheese

Directions:

1. Combine cucumber, onion and tomatoes in a large bowl.

2. Pour in the vinegar and toss to coat.

3. Cover and keep in the fridge until serving.

4. Stir in the cheese before you serve.

Nutrition Guide Per Serving:

Calories 101, Carbs 9g, Protein 4g, Fat 10g

Mushroom Stir Fry (Stove top)

Servings: 6

Prep Time: 10 minutes

Cook Time: 4 minutes

Ingredients:

1 1/2 pounds medium-size fresh mushrooms, halved

1/2 teaspoon dried Italian seasoning

2 garlic cloves, crushed

Salt and ground pepper

2 teaspoons lemon juice

Directions:

1. Spray cooking spray on a large skillet and place on medium heat.

2. Add the mushrooms, Italian seasoning and garlic. Season to taste with salt and pepper (about 1/4 teaspoon each should do).

3. Cook with constant stirring until mushrooms are tender and lightly browned, about 4 minutes.

4. Toss with lemon juice then serve.

Nutrition Guide Per Serving:

Calories 247, Carbs 7.3g, Protein 3.8g, Fat 24g

Cabbage Stir Fry (Stove top)
Very easy and very tasty.

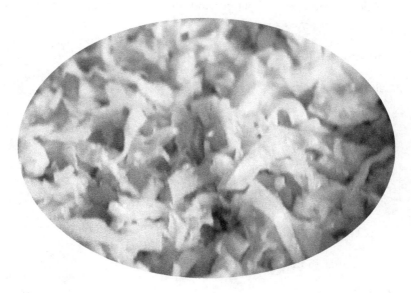

Servings: 6

Prep Time: 15 minutes

Cook Time: 5 minutes

Ingredients:

1/2 head red cabbage, chopped

3 tablespoons olive oil

2 small bell peppers, chopped

1/2 onion, chopped

Salt and ground black pepper, to taste

Directions:

1. Add the olive oil to a large skillet and place on high heat.

2. Add the cabbage, bell pepper and onion. Cook with constant stirring for 5 to 7 minutes then season to taste with salt and pepper.

Nutrition Guide Per Serving:

Calories 97, Carbs 8.3g, Protein 1.4g, Fat 7g

Zucchini Chips (Oven)

Servings: 4

Prep Time: 10 minutes

Cook Time: 25 minutes

Ingredients:

2 medium zucchinis, sliced

2 tablespoons of extra virgin olive oil

1/4 teaspoon black pepper

1/4 teaspoon salt

2 tablespoons of grated parmesan cheese

Directions:

1. Preheat your oven to 400°F. Place parchment paper on a sheet pan.

2. Brush zucchini slices on both sides with olive oil then arrange on the sheet pan in a single layer. Sprinkle with salt, pepper and cheese.

3. Bake until light brown on top, about 22-25 minutes.

Nutrition Guide Per Serving:

Calories 87, Carbs 2.5g, Protein 2.2g, Fat 7.7g

Sautéed Collard Greens (Stove top)

Servings: 4

Prep Time: 5 minutes

Cook Time: 12 minutes

Ingredients:

1 pound collard greens, chopped

2 tablespoons olive oil

4 garlic cloves, minced

Salt and pepper, to taste

Directions:

1. Add water to a large pot and bring to a boil. Add the collard greens, reduce the heat to simmer and cook for 5 minutes. Drain.

2. In a large saucepan, heat olive oil on medium heat. Cook the garlic with constant stirring for 1 minute. Add the collard greens, then sauté until tender, about 5 minutes.

3. Serve warm, sprinkled with salt and pepper

Nutrition Guide Per Serving:

Calories 97, Carbs 7g, Protein 3g, Fat 8g

Roasted Mushrooms And Asparagus (Oven)

Servings: 6

Prep Time: 10 minutes

Cook Time: 15 minutes

Ingredients:

1/2 pound fresh mushrooms, quartered

1 bunch fresh asparagus, trimmed

1/2 cup fresh basil, chopped

2 teaspoons olive oil

Kosher salt and freshly ground black pepper, to taste

Directions:

1. Preheat your oven to 450°F. Spray a sheet pan lightly with cooking spray.

2. In a bowl, combine mushrooms with asparagus and basil. Sprinkle with salt and pepper and drizzle with olive oil. Toss to coat then arrange on the prepared sheet pan.

3. Roast for about 15 minutes, or until the asparagus becomes tender.

Nutrition Guide Per Serving:

Calories 38, Carbs 4.6g, Protein 2.7g, Fat 1.9g

Roasted Tomato And Eggplant (Oven)

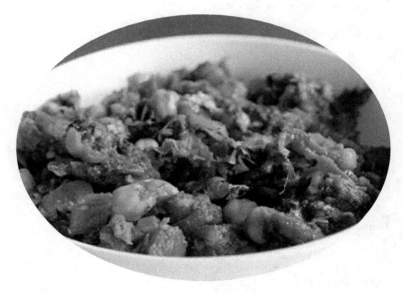

Servings: 4

Prep Time: 10 minutes

Cook Time: 15 minutes

Ingredients:

1 eggplant, sliced into rounds (1/2 inch thick)

1 large tomato, sliced

1/4 cup grated Parmesan cheese

Directions:

1. Preheat your oven to 400°F. Coat a baking sheet with cooking spray.

2. Place eggplant slices on the baking sheet and sprinkle with half of the Parmesan cheese. Arrange tomato slices on the eggplant and sprinkle with the remaining Parmesan.

3. Bake for about 12 to 15 minutes.

Nutrition Guide Per Serving:

Calories 66, Carbs 9.2g, Protein 3.4g, Fat 3g

Tomato Ginger Salad

Servings: 4

Prep Time: 10 minutes

Cook Time: minutes

Ingredients:

2 cups cherry tomatoes

1 tablespoon minced fresh ginger

2 tablespoons white vinegar

2 - 4 drops liquid Stevia

1/8 teaspoon salt

Directions:

1. In a bowl, mix together ginger, vinegar, Stevia and salt.

2. Add the tomatoes then gently toss to coat.

3. Cover and refrigerate until you want to serve.

Nutrition Guide Per Serving:

Calories 38, Carbs 8g, Protein 1g, Fat g

Easiest Roasted Salmon (Oven)

Servings: 4

Prep Time: 5 minutes

Cook Time: 15 minutes

Ingredients:

1 tablespoon olive oil

1 (1.5 pounds) center-cut salmon fillet

1/2 teaspoon of salt

1/4 teaspoon of pepper

Directions:

1. Preheat your oven to 350°F and place a rimmed baking pan in the oven.

2. Brush oil on the salmon and sprinkle all over with salt and pepper.

3. Remove the baking pan from the oven and place the fish in it, skin side down.

4. Bake until salmon easily flakes with a fork, about 15 to 18 minutes.

5. Cut into four even portions and serve.

Nutrition Guide Per Serving:

Calories 294, Carbs 0.2g, Protein 29g, Fat 19g

DESSERT / FAT BOMB

Peanut Butter Cookies (Oven)
Very low in carbs and as good as the real thing!

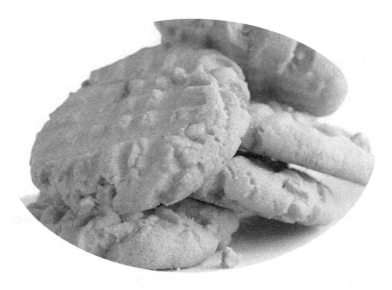

Servings: 16

Prep Time: 10 minutes

Cook Time: 12 minutes

Ingredients:

1 cup creamy peanut butter

1 egg

1 cup Splenda

1 teaspoon vanilla extract

Directions:

1. Preheat your oven to 350°F. Grease a cookie sheet.

2. Mix everything together in a medium bowl until well blended.

3. Roll the dough into small pieces, about the size of walnuts. Place on the cookie sheet.

4. Sprinkle the tops with a little splenda.

5. Cook for 12 minutes then transfer to a cooling rack. Dust with some more splenda and allow to cool. Transfer to an airtight container and refrigerate.

Nutrition Guide Per Serving:

Calories 96, Carbs 3g, Protein 4.3g, Fat 8.2g

Chocolate Peanut Butter Cookies (Oven)

Servings: 16

Prep Time: 10 minutes

Cook Time: 10minutes

Ingredients :

1 cup creamy peanut butter

2 tablespoons unsweetened cocoa powder

1 egg

1 tablespoon vanilla extract

1/4 cup Stevia sweetener

Directions:

1. Preheat your oven to 350°F.

2. In a food processor or mixer, mix together peanut butter, cocoa powder, egg, vanilla extract and Stevia sweetener.

3. Roll the dough into small balls, about 1 inch in diameter. Place on a baking sheet with about 1 inch in-between then use a fork to flatten each ball.

4. Bake for about 10 minutes, or until the edges are set.

5. Transfer cookies to a tray lined with parchment paper, let cool then refrigerate.

Nutrition Guide Per Serving:

Calories 107, Carbs 5.8g, Protein 4.4g, Fat 8.6g

Egg-Free Chocolate Mousse

Servings: 2

Prep Time: 5 minutes

Cook Time: minutes

Ingredients:

3 tablespoons cocoa powder

1 cup heavy whipping cream

2 packets Stevia

Directions:

1. Combine everything in a mixing bowl.

2. Mix until creamy and thickened.

3. Serve immediately.

Nutrition Guide Per Serving:

Calories 427, Carbs 7.5g, Protein 3g, Fat 44g

Coconut Balls Fat Bomb (Stove top)

A very sweet recipe that you can whip up very quickly.

Servings: 10

Prep Time: 1 hour 30 minutes

Cook Time: 5 minutes

Ingredients:

1 cup full fat coconut milk

1 cup coconut butter

1 teaspoon stevia powder extract

1 teaspoon vanilla extract

1 cup coconut flakes

Directions:

1. Combine coconut milk, coconut butter, stevia powder and vanilla extract in a double boiler. (Make a simple double boiler by adding a few inches of water to a saucepan and placing a heat proof glass bowl on the saucepan.)

2. Stir until the ingredients have melted and combined then remove from heat. Place the bowl in the refrigerator for at least 30 minutes for the mixture to harden.

3. Roll the mixture into 1-inch balls then roll each ball in coconut flakes.

4. Return to the refrigerate to chill for 1 hour before serving.

Nutrition Guide Per Serving:

Calories 340, Carbs 5.6g, Protein 3.5g, Fat 32g

Chocolate Fat Bombs (Stove top)

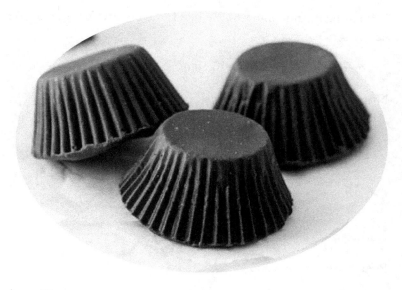

Servings: 12

Prep Time: 10 minutes

Cook Time: 10 minutes

Ingredients:

1/2 cup butter

1/2 cup almond butter

3 ounces 85% dark chocolate

1/4 teaspoon sea salt

1/4 cup swerve

Directions:

1. Combine all the ingredients in a double boiler. Heat and stir until melted and smooth.

2. Pour the mixture into silicone molds then freeze for 40 to 50 minutes before serving.

3. You can refrigerate for up to 10 days.

Nutrition Guide Per Serving:

Calories 95, Carbs 3g, Protein 1g, Fat 11g

Creamy Chocolate Frosty

Servings: 2

Prep Time: 5 minutes

Cook Time: minutes

Ingredients:

4 tablespoons heavy cream

1 cup water

4 tablespoons sugar free chocolate syrup

6 ice cubes

Directions:

1. Combine everything in a blender.

2. Process until frothy. Serve immediately.

Nutrition Guide Per Serving:

Calories 118, Carbs 4.9g, Protein 1.7g, Fat 11g

Keto Flan Cups (Oven)

Servings: 4

Prep Time: 10 minutes

Cook Time: 45 minutes

Ingredients:

2 large eggs

1/2 cup of water

1 cup heavy cream

1 teaspoon vanilla extract

1/4 cup sugar-free maple syrup

Directions:

1. Preheat your oven to 350°F. Add the eggs to a large bowl and whisk.

2. Add water, heavy cream, vanilla extract and maple syrup to a small skillet. Bring to a boil then remove from heat and whisk the mixture into the eggs.

3. Pour this mixture into four custard cups then place the cups in a large size roasting pan. Add hot water to the roasting pan up to halfway up the sides of the custard cups.

4. Bake until flans are set at the centers, about 35 to 40 minutes.

5. Remove from the oven, let cool for a few minutes then cover and place in the fridge until needed.

Nutrition Guide Per Serving:

Calories 248, Carbs 2.3g, Protein 4.5g, Fat 25g

Easy Chocolate Pudding

Servings: 4

Prep Time: 5 minutes

Cook Time: minutes

Ingredients:

1 tablespoon splenda sweetener

1 tablespoon unsweetened cocoa powder

2 teaspoons of vanilla extract

1/2 cup of heavy cream

Directions:

1. In a small bowl, mix together the cocoa powder, splenda and vanilla extract.

2. Whip the heavy cream until it has soft peaks.

3. Add the chocolate mixture and whip to combine.

4. Serve at once.

Nutrition Guide Per Serving:

Calories 115, Carbs 1.8g, Protein 1g, Fat 11.5g

Almond Butter Cookies (Oven)

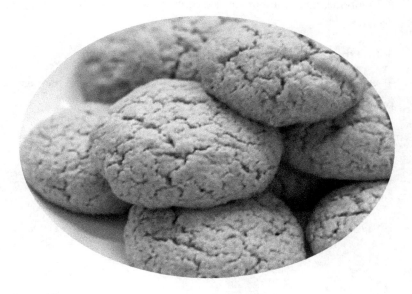

Servings: 12

Prep Time: 10 minutes

Cook Time: 12 minutes

Ingredients:

2 cups blanched almond flour

1 egg

1/2 cup butter, softened

1 teaspoon vanilla extract

1/2 cup Swerve sweetener

Directions:

1. Preheat your oven to 350°F. Place parchment paper on a baking sheet.

2. In a bowl, mix together all the ingredients until you have a well combined dough.

3. Roll the dough into 12 balls, about 1 inch in diameter.

4. Place on the baking sheet with about 1 inch in-between then use a fork to press down each ball.

5. Bake for 12 to 15 minutes or until golden around the edges.

Nutrition Guide Per Serving:

Calories 198, Carbs 11.7g, Protein 5g, Fat 19g

END

CPSIA information can be obtained
at www.ICGtesting.com
Printed in the USA
BVHW041214050519
547391BV00016B/615/P